Keto Chaffle

Appetizing Cookbook

2021

101 Affordable, Quick AND Easy and Mouthwatering
Sweet Ketogenic Recipes.

BY MEGAN FLOUR

Disclaimer

This publication is designed to provide competent and reliable information regarding the subject matter covered. However, it is sold with the understanding that the author
is not engaged in rendering professional or nutritional advice. Laws and practices often vary from state and country to country and if medical or other expert assistance is required, the services of a professional should be sought. The author specifically disclaims any liability that is
incurred from use or application of the content of this book.

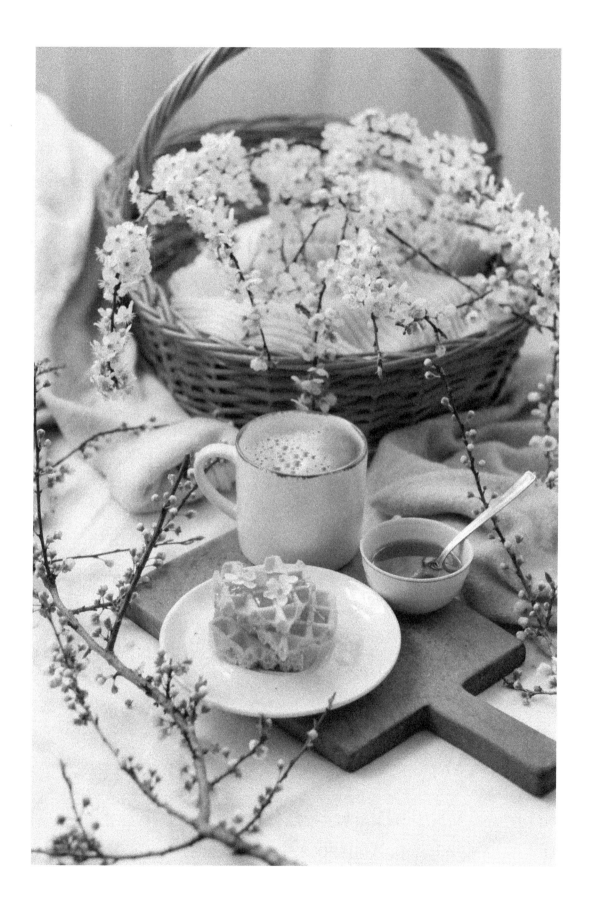

TABLE OF CONTENTS

WHY IS A CHAFFLE CALLED A CHAFFLE?

CHEESE+ WAFFLE= CHAFFLE!

IT'S A GREAT WAY TO EAT LOW CARB OR KETO FRIENDLY FOODS WITHOUT SACRIFICING TASTE.

Chaffles are a low-carb waffle they are called Chaffle because cheese is used as their base ingredient.

In just a few minutes, you can whip up a basic recipe with only two ingredients: eggs and cheese.

You can also customize your Chaffle, use a neutral cheese such as mozzarella or cream cheese, and apply your preferred keto sweetener to the batter before frying it. Whether blueberries or bananas, you can also use chocolate chips or low-sugar foods. For a delicious dessert of the Chaffle, finish with keto ice cream or keto whipped cream.

These keto waffles allow lower carbohydrate intake while fulfilling the nutrients needs of the person.

Chaffles become a popular snack of keto / low-carb. Using a waffle iron or a mini waffle machine, you can prepare a Chaffle. the cooking time is just a few minutes, so you end up with a warm, sweety, tasty bread / waffle substitute when you cook the Chaffle right.

You can also change the type of cheese you are using, resulting in major changes in the Chaffle's flavor and texture.

The two most popular options are cheddar cheese and mozzarella cheese, but you can also add parmesan cheese, cream cheese, or any other cheese that melts well.

Your Calories and net carb count will change a bit based on the cheese you use.

As usually, if you are using actual, whole milk cheese such as cheddar or mozzarella (as opposed to cream cheese or American cheese), it's absolutely carb-free.

Chaffle does not only include flour like a waffle but also different types of cheeses and egg and is simply a low-carb variety of a waffle. But they taste like waffles and are extremely healthy. They are also perfect for a ketogenic diet.

This book can be used to make the most delicious Chaffles ever.

CAN YOU FREEZE THE CHAFFLE?

Of course!

Any plastic you think is good in the freezer will work. Let it cool before putting it in the freezer because the heat and condensation make them sticky.

The best way to reheat them is to use a toaster, hot air container or pan in the oven.

Enjoy your meal!

HOW TO MAKE CHAFFLE?

BASIC SWEET CHAFFLES

Serving: 3
Preparation Time: 5 minutes
Cooking Time: 12 minutes

Ingredients:
- 1 large egg
- ½ cup grated Mozzarella cheese
- ¼ cup almond flour
- 1/8 teaspoon gluten-free baking powder
- 3 tablespoons Swerve

Direction
1. Preheat the mini waffle maker.
2. Using blender, mix all the ingredients and blend until smooth.
3. Scoop 1/3 of the batter into the preheated waffle maker.
4. Add them to the center as it spreads.
5. Close the waffle maker and cook for 2 to 4 minutes, checking the waffles after 2 minutes.
6. Keep an eye on the batter in case it overflows.
7. When done, open the lid and let cool down for 15 to 30 seconds.
8. The chaffle will firm up as it cools.
9. Use a spatula to transfer the chaffle onto a cooling rack gently.
10. Repeat with the remaining batter. When still warm, the chaffles will be soft.
11. They will crisp up when completely cooled.
12. Serve immediately or keep in a sealed container at room temperature for up to 3 days, or in the refrigerator for up to 1 week.

Nutrition:
- Calories:132
- Fat: 9.8g
- Protein: 8.4g

ALMOND BUTTER CHAFFLES

Servings: 2
Preparation Time: 5 minutes
Cooking Time: 10 minutes

Ingredients:
- 1 large organic egg, beaten
- 1/3 cup Mozzarella cheese, shredded
- 1 tablespoon Erythritol
- 2 tablespoons almond butter
- 1 teaspoon organic vanilla extract

Directions:
1. Preheat a mini waffle iron and then grease it.
2. In a medium bowl, place all ingredients and with a fork, mix until well combined.
3. Place half of the mixture into preheated waffle iron and cook for about 3-5 minutes or until golden brown.
4. Repeat with the remaining mixture.
5. Serve warm.

Nutrition:
- Calories: 153
- Net Carb: 2g
- Fat: 12.3g
- Carbohydrates: 3.6g
- Dietary Fiber: 1.6g
- Sugar: 1.2g
- Protein: 7.9g

BLUEBERRY KETO CHAFFLE

Serving: 5
Preparation Time: 5 minutes
Cooking Time: 17 minutes

Ingredients:
- 2 eggs
- 1 cup Mozzarella cheese
- 2 tablespoons almond flour
- 2 teaspoons Swerve
- 1 teaspoon baking powder
- 1 teaspoon cinnamon
- 3 tablespoon blueberries
- Nonstick cooking spray

Direction
1. Preheat the waffle maker.
2. Stir together the eggs, Mozzarella cheese, almond flour, Swerve, baking powder, cinnamon, and blueberries in a mixing bowl.
3. Brush the waffle maker with nonstick cooking spray.
4. Pour in a little bit less than ¼ a cup of blueberry waffle batter at a time.
5. Seal the lid and cook the chaffle for 3 to 5 minutes.
6. Check it at the 3-minute mark to see if it is crispy and brown.
7. If not or it sticks to the top of the waffle maker, close the lid and cook for an additional 1 to 2 minutes.
8. Serve sprinkled with additional Swerve.

Nutritions:
- Calories: 120
- Fat: 8.3g
- Protein: 8.4g

BRIE AND BLACKBERRY CHAFFLES

Servings: 2
Preparation time: 9 minutes
Cooking Time: 36 Minutes

Ingredients:
For the chaffles:
- 2 eggs, beaten
- 1 cup finely grated mozzarella cheese

For the topping:
- 1 ½ cups blackberries
- 1 lemon,
- 1 tsp zest and
- 2 tbsp juice
- 1 tbsp erythritol
- 4 slices Brie cheese

Directions:
For the chaffles:
1. Preheat the waffle iron.
2. Meanwhile, in a medium bowl, mix the eggs and mozzarella cheese.
3. Open the iron, pour in a quarter of the mixture, cover, and cook until crispy, 7 minutes.
4. Remove the chaffle onto a plate and make 3 more with the remaining batter.
5. Plate and set aside.
6. For the topping: In a medium pot, add the blackberries, lemon zest, lemon juice, and erythritol.
7. Cook until the blackberries and the sauce thickens, 5 minutes.
8. Turn the heat off.
9. Arrange the chaffles on the baking sheet and place two Brie cheese slices on each.
10. Top with blackberry mixture and transfer the baking sheet to the oven.
11. Bake until the cheese melts, 2 to 3 minutes.
12. Remove from the oven, allow cooling and serve afterward.

Nutrition:
- Calories 576

- Fats 42.22g
- Carbs 7.07g
- Net Carbs 3.67g
- Protein 42.35g

BUTTER CHAFLLES

Servings: 2
Preparation Time: 10 minutes
Cooking Time: 8 minutes

Ingredients:
- 2 tablespoons almond flour
- 1tablespoon coconut flour
- 1tablespoon Erythritol
- 1/2 teaspoon organic baking powder
- 1 organic egg
- 1 tablespoon butter, melted
- ½ teaspoon organic vanilla extract

Directions:
1. Preheat a mini waffle iron and then grease it.
2. In a bowl, place flours, Erythritol and baking powder and mix well.
3. Add the egg, butter and vanilla extract and beat until well combined.
4. Place half of the mixture into preheated waffle iron and cook for about 3-4 minutes or until golden brown.
5. Repeat with the remaining mixture.
6. Serve warm.

Nutrition
- Calories: 14g
- Net Carb: 1.9g
- Fat: 12.1g
- Carbohydrates: 4.2g
- Dietary Fiber: 2.3g
- Sugar: 0.6g
- Protein: 3.3g

BUTTER AND CREAM CHEESE CHAFFLES

Servings:4
Preparation Time: 10 minutes
Cooking Time: 16 minutes

Ingredients:
- 2 tablespoons butter, melted and cooled
- 2 large organic eggs
- 2 ounces cream cheese, softened
- 1/4 cup powdered Erythritol
- 1 teaspoons organic vanilla extract
- Pinch of salt
- 1/4 cup almond flour
- 2 tablespoons coconut flour
- 1 teaspoon organic baking powder

Directions:
1. Preheat a mini waffle iron and then grease it.
2. In a bowl, place the butter and eggs and beat until creamy.
3. Add the cream cheese, Erythritol, vanilla extract and salt and beat until well combined.
4. Add the flours and baking powder and beat until well combined.
5. Place 1/4 of the mixture into preheated waffle iron and cook for about 4 minutes or until golden brown.
6. Repeat with the remaining mixture.
7. Serve warm.

Nutrition:
- Calories: 202
- Net Carb: 2.8g
- Fat: 17.3g
- Carbohydrates: 5.1g
- Dietary Fiber: 2.3g
- Sugar: 0.7g
- Protein:4.8g

CACAO BUTTER CHAFFLES

Servings: 6
Preparation Time: 10 minutes
Cooking Time: 30 minutes

Ingredients:
- 2 organic egg whites
- ¼ cup butter, melted
- ¼ cup blanched almond flour
- ¼ cup cacao powder
- ¼ cup granulated Erythritol
- 2 teaspoons psyllium husk powder
- ½ teaspoon baking soda, sifted
- 1/8 teaspoon sea salt

Directions
1. Preheat a mini waffle iron and then grease it.
2. In a bowl, place all ingredients and beat until well combined.
3. Divide the mixture into 6 portions.
4. Place 1 portion of the mixture into preheated waffle iron and cook for about 3-5 minutes or until golden brown.
5. Repeat with the remaining mixture.
6. Serve warm.

Nutrition:
- Calories: 91
- Net Carb: 6.6g
- Fat: 9g
- Carbohydrates: 1g
- Dietary Fiber: 1.1g
- Sugar: 0.1g
- Protein: 2.3g

CACAO AND CHOCOLATE SYRUP CHAFFLES

Servings: 2
Preparation Time: 10 minutes
Cooking Time: 8 minutes

Ingredients:
- 1 large organic egg, beaten
- 1 ounce cream cheese, softened
- 1 tablespoon sugar-free chocolate syrup
- 1 tablespoon Erythritol
- ½ tablespoon cacao powder
- ¼ teaspoon organic baking powder
- ½ teaspoon organic vanilla extract

Directions:
1. Preheat a mini waffle iron and then grease it.
2. In a medium bowl, place all ingredients and with a fork, mix until well combined.
3. Place half of the mixture into preheated waffle iron and cook for about 3-4 minutes or until golden brown.
4. Repeat with the remaining mixture.
5. Serve warm.

Nutrition:
- Calories: 103
- Net Carb: 4.2g
- Fat: 7.7g
- Carbohydrates: 4.6g
- Dietary Fiber: 0.4g
- Sugar: 2g
- Protein: 4.5g

CACAO CREAM CHAFFLES

Servings: 2
Preparation Time: 10 minutes
Cooking Time: 10 minutes

Ingredients:
- 1 organic egg
- 1½ tablespoons cacao powder
- 2 tablespoons Erythritol
- 1 tablespoon heavy cream
- 1 teaspoon coconut flour
- ½ teaspoon organic baking powder
- ½ teaspoon organic vanilla extract
- ½ teaspoon powdered Erythritol

Directions:
1. Preheat a mini waffle iron and then grease it. In a bowl, place all ingredients except the powdered Erythritol and beat until well combined.
2. Place half of the mixture into preheated waffle iron and cook for about 3-5 minutes or until golden brown.
3. Repeat with the remaining mixture.
4. Serve warm with the sprinkling of powdered Erythritol.

Nutrition:
- Calories: 76
- Net Carb: 2.1g
- Fat: 5.9g
- Carbohydrates: 3.8g
- Dietary Fiber: 1.7g
- Sugar: 0.3g
- Protein: 3.8g

CACAO CREAM CHEESE CHAFFLES

Servings: 2
Preparation Time: 5 minutes
Cooking Time: 10 minutes

Ingredients:
- 1 organic egg 1 ounce cream cheese, softened
- 2 tablespoons almond flour
- 1 tablespoon cacao powder
- 2 teaspoons Erythritol
- 1 teaspoon organic vanilla extract

Directions:
1. Preheat a mini waffle iron and then grease it.
2. In a medium bowl, add all ingredients and with a fork, mix until well combined.
3. Place half of the mixture into preheated waffle iron and cook for about 3-5 minutes.
4. Repeat with the remaining mixture.
5. Serve warm.

Nutrition:
- Calories: 138
- Net Carb: 1.8g
- Fat: 11.4g
- Carbohydrates: 3.3g
- Dietary Fiber: 1.5g
- Sugar: 0.7g
- Protein: 4.3g

CACAO CREAM CHEESE CINNAMON CHAFFLES

Servings: 4
Preparation Time: 10 minutes
Cooking Time: 12 minutes

Ingredients:
- 2 ounces cream cheese, softened
- 1 organic egg
- 1 tablespoon coconut flour
- 2 teaspoon cacao powder
- 1½-2 tablespoons Erythritol
- 1 teaspoon organic vanilla extract
- ½ teaspoon baking soda
- 1 teaspoons ground cinnamon

Directions:
1. Preheat a mini waffle iron and then grease it.
2. In a medium bowl, add all ingredients and with a fork, mix until well combined.
3. Place ¼ of the mixture into preheated waffle iron and cook for about 3 minutes.
4. Repeat with the remaining mixture.
5. Serve warm.

Nutrition:
- Calories: 79
- Net Carb: 6.6g
- Fat: 6.4g
- Carbohydrates: 2.7g
- Dietary Fiber: 1.3g
- Sugar: 0.3g
- Protein: 2.9g

CACAO MOZZARELLA AND CREAM CHEESE CHAFFLES

Servings: 4
Preparation Time: 10 minutes
Cooking Time: 12 minutes

Ingredients:
- 1 large organic egg
- 1 large organic egg white
- ½ cup Mozzarella cheese, shredded
- 2 tablespoons cream cheese, softened
- 2 tablespoons coconut flour
- 2 tablespoons cacao powder
- 2 tablespoons granulated Erythritol
- ½ teaspoon organic baking powder

Directions:
1. Preheat a mini waffle iron and then grease it.
2. In a medium bowl, add all ingredients and with a fork, mix until well combined.
3. Place ¼ of the mixture into preheated waffle iron and cook for about 3 minutes.
4. Repeat with the remaining mixture.
5. Serve warm.

Nutrition:
- Calories: 71
- Net Carb: 2.2g
- Fat: 4.5g
- Carbohydrates: 4.5g
- Dietary Fiber: 2.3g
- Sugar: 0.2g
- Protein: 4.9g

Servings: 2
Preparation Time: 5 minutes
Cooking Time: 8 minutes

Ingredients:
- ½ cup Mozzarella cheese, shredded
- 1 medium organic egg
- 2 tablespoons almond meal
- 1 tablespoon cacao nibs
- 1 tablespoon granulated Erythritol
- 1 teaspoon organic vanilla extract

Directions:
1. Preheat a mini waffle iron and then grease it.
2. In a medium bowl, add all ingredients and with a fork, mix until well combined.
3. Place half of the mixture into preheated waffle iron and cook for about 2-4 minutes.
4. Repeat with the remaining mixture.
5. Serve warm.

Nutrition:
- Calories: 98
- Net Carb: 1.7g
- Fat: 6.9g
- Carbohydrates: 3.2g
- Dietary
- Fiber: 1.5g
- Sugar: 0.7g
- Protein: 6.5g

CACAO WHIPPING CREAM CHAFFLES

Servings: 2
Preparation Time: 10 minutes
Cooking Time: 8 minutes

Ingredients:
- 1 tablespoon almond flour
- 2 tablespoons cacao powder
- 2 tablespoons granulated Erythritol
- ¼ teaspoon organic baking powder
- 1 organic egg
- 1 tablespoon heavy whipping cream
- ¼ teaspoon organic vanilla extract
- 1/8 teaspoon organic almond extract

Directions:
1. Preheat a mini waffle iron and then grease it.
2. In a bowl, place all ingredients and beat until well combined.
3. Place half of the mixture into preheated waffle iron and cook for about 4 minutes or until golden brown.
4. Repeat with the remaining mixture.
5. Serve warm.

Nutrition:
- Calories: 94
- Net Carb: 2g
- Fat: 7.9g
- Carbohydrates: 3.9g
- Dietary Fiber: 1.9g
- Sugar: 0.4g
- Protein: 3.9g

CEREAL CHAFFLE CAKE

Servings: 3
Preparation time: 10 minutes
Cooking Time: 8 Minutes

Ingredients:
- 1 egg
- 2 tablespoons almond flour
- ½ teaspoon coconut flour
- 1 tablespoon melted butter
- 1 tablespoon cream cheese
- 1 tablespoon plain cereal, crushed
- ¼ teaspoon vanilla extract
- ù¼ teaspoon baking powder
- 1 tablespoon sweetener
- 1/8 teaspoon xanthan gum

Directions:
1. Plug in your waffle maker to preheat.
2. Add all the ingredients in a large bowl.
3. Mix until well blended.
4. Let the batter rest for 2 minutes before cooking.
5. Pour half of the mixture into the waffle maker.
6. Seal and cook for 4 minutes.
7. Make the next chaffle using the same steps.

Nutrition:
- Calories: 154
- Total Fat: 21.2g
- Saturated Fat: 10 g
- Cholesterol: 113.3mg
- Sodium: 96.9mg
- Potassium: 453 mg
- Total Carbohydrate: 5.9g
- Dietary Fiber: 1.7g
- Protein: 4.6g
- Total Sugars: 2.7g

CHAFFLED BROWNIE SUNDAE

Servings: 2
Preparation time: 9 minutes
Cooking Time: 30 Minutes

Ingredients:
For the chaffles:
- 2 eggs, beaten
- 1 tbsp unsweetened cocoa powder
- 1 tbsp erythritol
- 1 cup finely grated mozzarella cheese

For the topping:
- 3 tbsp unsweetened chocolate, chopped
- 3 tbsp unsalted butter
- ½ cup swerve sugar Low-carb ice cream for topping
- 1 cup whipped cream for topping
- 3 tbsp sugar-free caramel sauce

Directions:
For the chaffles:
1. Preheat the waffle iron.
2. Meanwhile, in a medium bowl, mix all the ingredients for the chaffles.
3. Open the iron, pour in a quarter of the mixture, cover, and cook until crispy, 7 minutes.
4. Remove the chaffle onto a plate and make 3 more with the remaining batter.
5. Plate and set aside.

For the topping:
- Meanwhile, melt the chocolate and butter in a medium saucepan with occasional stirring, 2 minutes.

To Servings:
1. Divide the chaffles into wedges and top with the ice cream, whipped cream, and swirl the chocolate sauce and caramel sauce on top.
2. Serve immediately.

Nutrition:
- Calories 165
- Fats 11.39g
- Carbs 3.81g
- Net Carbs 2.91g
- Protein 79g

CHAFFLE CANNOLI

Servings: 2
Preparation time: 9 minutes
Cooking Time: 28 Minutes

Ingredients:
For the chaffles:
- 1 large egg
- 1 egg yolk
- 3 tbsp butter, melted
- 1 tbsp swerve confectioner's
- 1 cup finely grated Parmesan cheese
- 2 tbsp finely grated mozzarella cheese

For the cannoli filling:
- ½ cup ricotta cheese
- 2 tbsp swerve confectioner's sugar
- 1 tsp vanilla extract
- 2 tbsp unsweetened chocolate chips for garnishing

Directions:
1. Preheat the waffle iron.
2. Meanwhile, in a medium bowl, mix all the ingredients for the chaffles.
3. Open the iron, pour in a quarter of the mixture, cover, and cook until crispy, 7 minutes.
4. Remove the chaffle onto a plate and make 3 more with the remaining batter.
5. Meanwhile, for the cannoli filling: Beat the ricotta cheese and swerve confectioner's sugar until smooth.
6. Mix in the vanilla.
7. On each chaffle, spread some of the filling and wrap over.
8. Garnish the creamy ends with some chocolate chips.
9. Serve immediately.

Nutrition:
- Calories 308
- Fats 25.05g
- Carbs 5.17g

- Net Carbs 5.17g
- Protein 15.18g

CHAFFLES WITH KETO ICE CREAM

Servings: 2
Preparation time: 10 minutes
Cooking Time: 14 Minutes

Ingredients:
- 1 egg, beaten
- ½ cup finely grated mozzarella cheese
- ¼ cup almond flour
- 2 tbsp swerve confectioner's sugar
- 1/8 tsp xanthan gum Low-carb ice cream (flavor of your choice) for serving

Directions:
1. Preheat the waffle iron.
2. In a medium bowl, mix all the ingredients except the ice cream.
3. Open the iron and add half of the mixture.
4. Close and cook until crispy, 7 minutes.
5. Transfer the chaffle to a plate and make second one with the remaining batter.
6. On each chaffle, add a scoop of low carb ice cream, fold into half-moons.
7. Serve

Nutrition
- Calories 89
- Fats 48g
- Carbs 1.67g
- Net Carbs 1.37g
- Protein 5.91g 3.

CHAFFLES WITH RASPBERRY SYRUP

Servings: 2
Preparation time: 9 minutes
Cooking Time: 38 Minutes

Ingredients:
For the chaffles:
- 1 egg, beaten
- ½ cup finely shredded cheddar cheese
- 1 tsp almond flour
- 1 tsp sour cream

For the raspberry syrup:
- 1 cup fresh raspberries
- ¼ cup swerve sugar
- ¼ cup water
- 1 tsp vanilla extract

Directions:
For the chaffles:
1. Preheat the waffle iron.
2. Meanwhile, in a medium bowl, mix the egg, cheddar cheese, almond flour, and sour cream.
3. Open the iron, pour in half of the mixture, cover, and cook until crispy, 7 minutes.
4. Remove the chaffle onto a plate and make another with the remaining batter.

For the raspberry syrup:
1. Meanwhile, add the raspberries, swerve sugar, water, and vanilla extract to a medium pot.
2. Set over low heat and cook until the raspberries soften and sugar becomes syrupy.
3. Occasionally stir while mashing the raspberries as you go.
4. Turn the heat off when your desired consistency is achieved and set aside to cool.
5. Drizzle some syrup on the chaffles and enjoy when ready.

Nutrition:
- Calories 105
- Fats 7.11g

- Carbs 4.31g
- Net Carbs 2.21g
- Protein 5.83g

CHAFFLE TORTILLA

Servings: 2
Cooking Time: 8 Minutes

Ingredients:

- 1 egg
- 1/2 cup cheddar cheese, shredded
- 1 teaspoon baking powder
- 4 tablespoons almond flour
- 1/4 teaspoon garlic powder
- 1 tablespoon almond milk
- Homemade salsa
- Sour cream
- Jalapeno pepper, chopped

Directions:

1. Preheat your waffle maker.
2. Beat the egg in a bowl.
3. Stir in the cheese, baking powder, flour, garlic powder and almond milk.
4. Pour half of the batter into the waffle maker.
5. Cover and cook for 4 minutes.
6. Open and transfer to a plate. Let cool for 2 minutes.
7. Do the same for the remaining batter.
8. Top the waffle with salsa, sour cream and jalapeno pepper.
9. Roll the waffle.

Nutrition:

- Calories 225
- Total Fat 17.6g
- Saturated Fat 9.99
- Cholesterol 117Ing
- Sodium 367mg
- Potassium 366mg
- Total Carbohydrate 6g
- Dietary Fiber 0.8g
- Protein 11.3g
- Total Sugars 1.9g

CHOCOLATE CHAFFLES

Servings: 2
Prep Time: 3 minutes
Cook Time: 10 minutes

Ingredients
- ¾ cup shredded mozzarella
- 1 large egg
- 2 Tbsp almond flour
- 2 Tbsp allulose
- ½ Tbsp melted butter
- 1½ Tbsp cocoa powder
- ½ tsp vanilla extract
- ½ tsp psyllium husk powder
- ¼ tsp baking powder

Directions
1. Turn on waffle maker to heat and oil it with cooking spray.
2. Mix all ingredients in a small bowl.
3. Pour ¼ cup batter into a 4-inch waffle maker.
4. Cook for 2-3 minutes, or until crispy.
5. Transfer chaffle to a plate and set aside.
6. Repeat with remaining batter.

Nutritional Value (per serving):
- Calories: 293
- Fat: 24 g
- Carbohydrate: 8g
- Protein: 15g

CHOCOLATE AND ALMOND CHAFFLE

Servings: 2
Preparation time: 6 minutes
Cooking Time: 12 Minutes

Ingredients:
- 1 egg
- ¼ cup mozzarella cheese, shredded
- 1 oz. cream cheese
- 2 teaspoons sweetener 1 teaspoon vanilla
- 2 tablespoons cocoa powder
- 1 teaspoon baking powder
- 2 tablespoons almonds, chopped
- 4 tablespoons almond flour

Directions:
1. Blend all the ingredients in a bowl while the waffle maker is preheating.
2. Pour some of the mixture into the waffle maker.
3. Close and cook for 4 minutes.
4. Transfer the chaffle to a plate.
5. Let cool for 2 minutes.
6. Repeat steps using the remaining mixture.

Nutrition:
- Calories: 1
- Total Fat:13.1g
- Saturated Fat: 5g
- Cholesterol: 99mg
- Sodium: 99mg
- Potassium: 481mg
- Total Carbohydrate: 9.1g
- Dietary Fiber: 3.8g
- Protein: 7.8g
- Total Sugars 0.8g

CHOCOLATE CAKE WITH ALMOND BUTTER

Servings: 12
Preparation time: 15 minutes
Cooking time: 10 minutes

Ingredients:
- 1 cup of almond butter
- 3/4 cup powdered erythritol
- 3 large eggs
- 10 tablespoons of cocoa powder
- 1/2 teaspoon baking powder

Directions
1. Using a food processor, blend the almond butter and erythritol.
2. Then add the eggs, cocoa powder, baking powder and a pinch of salt.
3. Transfer the dough onto a greased 23 cm × 23 cm baking sheet and smooth the tabletop with the spatula.
4. Bake for 10 minutes at 160 ° C.
5. Allow the dough to cool completely before slicing.
6. Enjoy!

Nutrition:
- Fat: 56% (14 g)
- Protein: 32% (8 g)
- Net carbohydrates: 12% (3 g)
- kcal: 153

CHOCOLATE CHIPS CINNAMON CHAFFLES

Servings: 2
Preparation Time: 10 minutes
Cooking Time: 8 minutes

Ingredients:
- 1 organic egg
- ½ cup Mozzarella cheese, shredded
- 1 tablespoon almond flour
- 2 tablespoons 70% dark chocolate chips
- ½ tablespoon granulated Erythritol
- ¼ teaspoon ground cinnamon

Directions:
1. Preheat a mini waffle iron and then grease it.
2. In a medium bowl, place all ingredients and with a fork, mix until well combined.
3. Place half of the mixture into preheated waffle iron and cook for about 4 minutes or until golden brown.
4. Repeat with the remaining mixture.
5. Serve warm.

Nutrition:
- Calories: 110
- Net Carb: 5.5g
- Fat: 7.3g
- Carbohydrates: 6g
- Dietary Fiber: 0.5g
- Sugar: 4.3g
- Protein: 5.3g

CHOCOLATE CHIPS MAYONNAISE CHAFFLES

Servings: 6
Preparation Time: 10 minutes
Cooking Time: 30 minutes

Ingredients:
- 4 tablespoons mayonnaise
- 4 organic eggs
- 2 tablespoons Erythritol
- ¼ cup coconut flour
- ½ tablespoon organic baking powder
- ½ teaspoon organic vanilla extract
- ¼ cup 70% dark chocolate chips

Directions
1. Preheat a mini waffle iron and then grease it.
2. In a bowl, place all ingredients and beat until well combined.
3. Divide the mixture into 6 portions.
4. Place 1 portion of the mixture into preheated waffle iron and cook for about 4-5 minutes or until golden brown.
5. Repeat with the remaining mixture.
6. Serve warm.

Nutrition:
- Calories: 191
- Net Carb: 3.5g
- Fat: 15.4g
- Carbohydrates: 6.9g
- Dietary Fiber: 3.4g
- Sugar: 0.3g
- Protein: 5.7g

CHOCOLATE MELT CHAFFLES

Servings: 2
Preparation time: 9 minutes
Cooking Time: 36 Minutes

Ingredients:

For the chaffles:
- 2 eggs, beaten
- ¼ cup finely grated Gruyere cheese
- 2 tbsp heavy cream
- 1 tbsp coconut flour
- 2 tbsp cream cheese, softened
- 3 tbsp unsweetened cocoa powder
- 2 tsp vanilla extract
- A pinch of salt

For the chocolate sauce:
- 1/3 cup + 1 tbsp heavy cream
- 1 ½ oz unsweetened baking chocolate, chopped
- 1 ½ tsp sugar-free maple syrup
- 1 ½ tsp vanilla extract

Directions:

For the chaffles:
1. Preheat the waffle iron.
2. In a medium bowl, mix all the ingredients for the chaffles.
3. Open the iron and add a quarter of the mixture.
4. Close and cook until crispy, 7 minutes.
5. Transfer the chaffle to a plate and make 3 more with the remaining batter.

For the chocolate sauce:
1. Pour the heavy cream into saucepan and simmer over low heat, 3 minutes.
2. Turn the heat off and add the chocolate.
3. Allow melting for a few minutes and stir until fully melted, 5 minutes.
4. Mix in the maple syrup and vanilla extract.

5. Assemble the chaffles in layers with the chocolate sauce sandwiched between each layer.
6. Slice and serve immediately.

Nutrition:
- Calories 172
- Fats 13.57g
- Carbs 6.65g
- Net Carbs 3.65g
- Protein 5.76g

CHOCOLATY STRAWBERRY CHAFFLES

Servings: 3
Preparation Time: 10 minutes
Cooking Time: 13½ minutes

Ingredients:
- ½ cup Mozzarella cheese shredded
- 1 ounce cream cheese, softened
- 2 tablespoon almond flour
- 3 tablespoon powdered Erythritol
- 1 large organic egg
- 2 tablespoon heavy whipping cream
- ½ teaspoon vanilla extract
- 2-3 fresh strawberries, hulled and smashed
- 1 tablespoon cacao powder

Diretions:
1. Preheat a mini waffle iron and then grease it.
2. In a microwave-safe bowl, add the Mozzarella and cream cheeses and microwave for about 1-1½ minutes or until melted completely, stirring after every 30 seconds.
3. Add the almond flour and Erythritol and with your hands, knead until well combined.
4. Add the egg, whipping cream and vanilla extract and beat until smooth.
5. Add the strawberries and cacao powder and stir to combine.
6. Place1/3 of the mixture into preheated waffle iron and cook for about 3-4 minutes or until golden brown.
7. Repeat with the remaining mixture.
8. Serve warm.

Nutrition:
- Calories: 143
- Net Carb: 2g
- Fat: 12.3g
- Carbohydrates: 3.2g
- Dietary Fiber: 1.2g
- Sugar: 0.8g
- Protein: 4.7g

CHOCOLATY PUMPKIN CHAFFLES

Servings: 3
Preparation Time: 10 minutes
Cooking Time: 12 minutes

Ingredients:
- 1 organic egg
- 4 teaspoons homemade pumpkin puree
- ½ cup Mozzarella cheese, shredded
- 1 tablespoon almond flour
- 2 tablespoons granulated Erythritol
- ¼ teaspoon pumpkin pie spice
- 4 teaspoons 70% dark chocolate chips

Instructions:
1. In a bowl, place the egg and pumpkin puree and mix well.
2. Add the remaining ingredients except for chocolate chips and mix until well combined.
3. Gently, fold in the chocolate chips and lemon zest.
4. Place 1/3 of the mixture into preheated waffle iron and cook for about 4 minutes or until golden brown.
5. Repeat with the remaining mixture.
6. Serve warm.

Nutrition:
- Calories: 97
- Net Carb: 1.9g
- Fat: 7.1g
- Carbohydrates: 1.4g
- Dietary Fiber: 2.6g
- Sugar: 0.4g
- Protein: 4.2g

CHOCOLATE CHIPS PEANUT BUTTER CHAFFLES

Servings: 2
Preparation Time: 10 minutes
Cooking Time: 8 minutes

Ingredients:
- 1 organic egg, beaten
- ¼ cup Mozzarella cheese, shredded
- 2 tablespoons creamy peanut butter
- 1 tablespoon almond flour
- 1 tablespoon granulated Erythritol
- 1 teaspoon organic vanilla extract
- 1 tablespoon 70% dark chocolate chips

Directions:
1. Preheat a mini waffle iron and then grease it.
2. In a bowl, place all ingredients except chocolate chips and beat until well combined.
3. Gently, fold in the chocolate chips.
4. Place half of the mixture into preheated waffle iron and cook for about 4 minutes or until golden brown.
5. Repeat with the remaining mixture. Serve warm.

Nutrition:
- Calories: 214
- Net Carb: 4.1g
- Fat: 16.8g
- Carbohydrates: 6.4g
- Dietary Fiber: 2.3g
- Sugar: 2.1g
- Protein: 8.8g

CHOCOLATE CHIPS LEMON CHAFFLES

Servings: 4
Preparation Time: 10 minutes
Cooking Time: 8 minutes
Ingredients:
- 2 organic eggs
- ½ cup Mozzarella cheese, shredded
- ¾ teaspoon organic lemon extract
- ½ teaspoon organic vanilla extract
- 2 teaspoons Erythritol
- ½ teaspoon psyllium husk powder Pinch of salt
- 1 tablespoon 70% dark chocolate chips
- ¼ teaspoon lemon zest, grated finely

Directions:
1. Preheat a mini waffle iron and then grease it.
2. In a bowl, place all ingredients except for chocolate chips and lemon zest and beat until well combined.
3. Gently, fold in the chocolate chips and lemon zest.
4. Place ¼ of the mixture into preheated waffle iron and cook for about 4 minutes or until golden brown.
5. Repeat with the remaining mixture.
6. Serve warm.

Nutritional Information
- Calories: 71
- Net Carb: 1g
- Fat: 4.8g
- Carbohydrates: 1.5g
- Dietary Fiber: 0.5g
- Sugar: 0.3g
- Protein: 4.3g

CHOCOLATE CHIPS WHIPPING CREAM CHAFFLES

Servings: 2
Preparation Time: 10 minutes
Cooking Time: 8 minutes

Ingredients:
- 1 organic egg
- 1 tablespoon heavy whipping cream
- ½ teaspoon coconut flour
- 1¾ teaspoons monk-fruit sweetener
- ¼ teaspoon organic baking powder
- Pinch of salt
- 1 tablespoon 70% dark chocolate chips

Directions
1. Preheat a mini waffle iron and then grease it.
2. In a bowl, place all ingredients except for chocolate chips and beat until well combined.
3. Fold in the blackberries.
4. Place half of the mixture into preheated waffle iron and top with half of the chocolate chips.
5. Cook for about 3-4 minutes or until golden brown.
6. Repeat with the remaining mixture and chocolate chips.
7. Serve warm.

Nutrition:
- Calories: 110
- Net Carb: 1.8g
- Fat: 9g
- Carbohydrates: 3.1g
- Dietary Fiber: 1.3g
- Sugar: 0.2g
- Protein: 4g

CHOCOLATE TRUFFLES

Servings: 10
Preparation time: 25 minutes
Cooking time: 0 minutes

Ingredients:
- 1/2 cup of fondant
- 110 g of dark chocolate
- 2 teaspoons of unsalted butter
- 1/2 cup of granulated erythritol
- 1 teaspoon of sea salt in flakes

Directions:
1. Heat the cream in a water bath until hot
2. Cut the chocolate into small pieces and add them to the hot fondant.
3. Stir until chocolate melts.
4. Take the pot off the oven, add and mix the butter.
5. Then add erythritol, mix and refrigerate for an hour.
6. Using the ice cream scoop, take a ball of approximately 2.5 cm and round it with lightly oiled fingers.
7. Place the balls on a parchment-lined plate and decorate with sea salt flakes.
8. Put in the fridge for 1-2 hours and enjoy delicious truffles!

Nutrition:
- Fat: 80% (10 g)
- Protein: 12% (1.5 g)
- Net carbohydrates: 8% (1 g)
- kcal: 110

CINNAMON CHAFFLES

Servings: 2
Preparation Time: 5 minutes
Cooking Time: 8 minutes

Ingredients:
- ½ cup Mozzarella cheese, shredded
- 1 medium organic egg
- 1 tablespoon almond flour
- 1 tablespoon Erythritol
- 2 teaspoons ground cinnamon
- 1 teaspoon organic vanilla extract

Directions:
1. Preheat a mini waffle iron and then grease it.
2. In a medium bowl, place all ingredients and with a fork, mix until well combined.
3. Place ¼ of the mixture into preheated waffle iron and cook for about 3-4 minutes or until golden brown.
4. Repeat with the remaining mixture.
5. Serve warm.

Nutrition:
- Calories: 166
- Net Carb: 2.3g
- Fat: 12.1g
- Carbohydrates: 3.9g
- Dietary Fiber: 1.6g
- Sugar: 0.6g
- Protein: 9.9g

CINNAMON ROLL CHAFFLE

Servings: 3
Cooking Time: 9 Minutes

Ingredients:
- 1 egg (beaten)
- 1/2 cup shredded mozzarella cheese
- 1 tsp cinnamon
- 1 tsp sugar free maple syrup
- 1/4 tsp baking powder
- 1 tbsp almond flour
- 1/2 tsp vanilla extract

Topping:
- 2 tsp granulated swerve
- 1 tbsp heavy cream
- 4 tbsp cream cheese

Directions:
1. Plug the waffle maker to preheat it and spray it with a non-stick spray.
2. In a mixing bowl, whisk together the egg, maple syrup and vanilla extract
3. In another mixing bowl, combine the cinnamon, almond flour, baking powder and mozzarella cheese.
4. Pour in the egg mixture into the flour mixture and mix until the Ingredients are well combined.
5. Pour in an appropriate amount of the batter into the waffle maker and spread out the batter to the edges to cover all the holes on the waffle maker.
6. Close the waffle maker and bake for about 3 minute or according to your waffle maker's settings.
7. After the cooking cycle, use a silicone or plastic utensil to remove the chaffle from the waffle maker.
8. Repeat step 5 to 7 until you have cooked all the batter into chaffles
9. For the TOPPING, combine the cream cheese, swerve and heavy cream in a microwave safe dish.
10. Place the dish in a microwave and microwave on high until the mixture is melted and smooth.
11. Stir every 15 seconds

12. Top the chaffles with the cream mixture and enjoy.

Nutrition:
- Fat 9.99 13%
- Carbohydrate 3.8g 1%
- Sugars 0.3g
- Protein 4.8g

CINNAMON ROLL KETO CHAFFLES

Servings: 3
Cooking Time: 10 Minutes

Ingredients:
Cinnamon Roll Chaffle
- 1/2 cup mozzarella cheese
- 1 tablespoon almond flour
- 1/4 tsp baking powder
- 1 egg
- 1 tsp cinnamon
- 1 tsp Granulated Swerve

Cinnamon Roll Swirl
- 1 tbsp butter
- 1 tsp cinnamon
- 2 tsp confectioners Swerve

Keto Cinnamon Roll Glaze
- 1 tablespoon butter
- 1 tablespoon cream cheese
- 1/4 tsp vanilla extract
- 2 tsp Swerve confectioners

Directions:
1. Plug in your Mini Dash Waffle maker and let it heat up.
2. In a small bowl mix the mozzarella cheese, almond flour, baking powder, egg, 1 teaspoon cinnamon, and 1 teaspoon swerve granulated and set aside.
3. In another small bowl, add a tablespoon of butter, 1 teaspoon cinnamon, and 2 teaspoons of Swerve confectioners sweetener.
4. Microwave for 15 seconds and mix well
5. Spray the waffle maker with nonstick spray and add 1/3 of the batter to your waffle maker. Swirl in 1/3 of the cinnamon, swerve, and butter mixture onto the top of it.
6. Close the waffle maker and let cook for 3-4 minutes.
7. When the first cinnamon roll chaffle is done, make the second and then make the third.
8. While the third chaffle is cooking place 1 tablespoon butter and 1 tablespoon of cream cheese in a small bowl.
9. Heat in the microwave for 10-15 seconds.

10. Start at 10, and if the cream cheese is not soft enough to mix with the butter heat for an additional 5 seconds.
11. Add the vanilla extract, and the Swerve confectioner sweetener to the butter and cream cheese and mix well using a whisk.
12. Drizzle keto cream cheese glaze on top of chaffle.

Nutrition:(per serving):
- Calories: 180 kcal;
- Carbohydrates: 3g;
- Protein: 79;
- Fat: 16g;
- Saturated Fat:9g;
- Cholesterol: 95mg;
- Sodium:221mg ;
- Potassium: 77 mg;
- Fiber: 1 g;
- Sugar: 1g:
- Vitamin A: 505 IU;
- Calcium: 148 mg;
- Iron: 1mg

COCONUT CAKE WITHOUT SUGAR

Servings: 8
Preparation time: 30 minutes
Cooking time: 15 minutes |

Ingredients:
- 200 g of unsweetened coconut flakes
- 40 g of coconut oil, melted
- 60 g of powdered erythritol
- 2 g xanthan gum
- 480 g cream 36%

Directions:
1. Blend 110 g of coconut flakes, coconut oil and 15 g of erythritol.
2. Put the mixture on the bottom of a 20 cm diameter pan and knead well.
3. Bake for 10 minutes at 175 ° C - be careful, it can burn quickly.
4. Mix the cream with the xanthan gum and heat it in a pot over low heat until the ingredients combine well.
5. Then add the remaining powdered erythritol and 60 g of coconut flakes.
6. Bring to a boil, then wait 10 minutes.
7. On a baking sheet, toast 30 g of coconut flakes for 5 minutes at 175 ° C.
8. They will be needed to sprinkle the dough.
9. Pour the cream mixture onto the baked and cooled bottom of the cake.
10. Sprinkle with roasted coconut and refrigerate until solid.
11. Enjoy your meal!

Nutrition:
- Fat: 42.5 g
- Protein: 3.5 g
- Net carbohydrates: 7.5 g
- kcal: 413

COTTAGE CHEESE CHAFFLES

Servings: 4
Preparation Time: 10 minutes
Cooking Time: 0 minutes

Ingredients:
- 1cup almond flour
- 2 tablespoons Erythritol
- ¼ cup cottage cheese
- ¼ cup unsweetened almond milk
- 2 organic eggs
- ½ teaspoon organic baking powder
- ½ teaspoon organic almond extract

Directions:
1. Preheat a waffle iron and then grease it.
2. In a high-speed blender, add all ingredients and pulse until well combined and smooth.
3. Place ¼ of the mixture into preheated waffle iron and cook for about 3-5 minutes or until golden brown.
4. Repeat with the remaining mixture.
5. Serve warm.

Nutrition:
- Calories: 229
- Net Carb: 3.1g
- Fat: 17.7g
- Carbohydrates: 6.2g
- Dietary Fiber: 3.1g
- Sugar: 1.3g
- Protein:4.8g

CRANBERRY SWIRL CHAFFLE

Servings: 2
Cooking Time: 25 minutes

Ingredients
For the Cranberry Sauce:
- Two tablespoons of erythritol (granulated)
- Half a cup each of Water
- Cranberries (frozen or fresh)
- Half a teaspoon of vanilla extract

For the Chaffles:
- One oz. of cream cheese (must be kept at room temperature)
- One egg
- A quarter teaspoon of baking powder
- One teaspoon of coconut flour
- Half a teaspoon of vanilla extract
- One tablespoon of Swerve

For the Frosting:
- One tablespoon each of Swerve Butter (kept at room temperature)
- One oz. of cream cheese (kept at room temperature)
- Orange zest (grated)
- One-eighth teaspoon of orange extract

Directions:
For the cranberry swirl,
1. Take a medium-sized saucepan and, in it, add water, cranberries, and erythritol.
2. Combine all the ingredients well and gradually bring them to a boil.
3. Once the mixture starts to boil, allow them to simmer for a while.
4. Continue simmering for about ten to fifteen minutes.
5. By this time, the sauce will start to thicken, and the cranberries will pop.
6. Once done, remove the saucepan from the heat and add the vanilla extract.
7. Stir it in.
8. Use a spoon (specifically, the back of the spoon) to mash the cranberries properly, and this will give the sauce a chunky consistency.

9. When you bring the saucepan off the heat, you will notice that the sauce thickens considerably.

For the chaffles,
1. Start by heating your waffle iron, and before you put the batter in it, you have to make sure that it is thoroughly heated.
2. Now, take all the ingredients of the chaffle and add them to a medium-sized bowl.
3. Whisk them well.
4. Take two tablespoons of the batter at a time and add them to the waffle iron.
5. Once you have added the batter, take half a portion of the cranberry sauce that you just prepared and add it over the batter in small dollops.
6. Close the iron and cook the chaffle for about five minutes.
7. Once it is done, remove the chaffle and place it on a wire rack.
8. Do the same for the second chaffle.

For the frosting,
1. Take all the ingredients required for the frosting apart from the orange zest and add them to a bowl.
2. Whisk them well so that you get a smooth consistency.
3. Now, you simply have to spread this frosting over the chaffles.
4. Once you have applied the frosting, sprinkle the grated orange zest on top.

Nutrition:
- Calories: 70 |
- Carb: 4.9g |
- Protein: 1.8g |
- Fat: 6g

CREAM CHEESE CHAFFLES

Servings:4
Preparation Time: 5 minutes
Cooking Time: 8 minutes

Ingredients:
- 2 organic eggs
- 2 ounces cream cheese, softened
- 4-5 drops liquid stevia

Directions:
1. Preheat a waffle iron and then grease it.
2. In a high-speed blender, add all ingredients and pulse until well combined and smooth.
3. Place 1/4 of the mixture into preheated waffle iron and cook for about 3-4 minutes or until golden brown.
4. Repeat with the remaining mixture.
5. Serve warm.

Nutrition:
- Calories: 81
- Net Carb: 0.6g
- Fat: 7.1g
- Carbohydrates: 0.6g
- Sugar: 0.2g
- Protein: 3.8g

CREAM CHEESE AND BUTTER CHAFFLES

Servings: 4
Preparation Time: 10 minutes
Cooking Time: 16 minutes

Ingredients:

2 large organic eggs
2 ounces cream cheese, softened
1tablespoon butter, melted
1/2 teaspoon organic vanilla extract
1/4 cup almond flour
1/2 tablespoon Erythritol
1/2 teaspoon organic baking powder

Directions:

1. Preheat a mini waffle iron and then grease it.
2. In a bowl, place flour, Erythritol and baking powder and mix well.
3. Add the egg, cream cheese and vanilla extract and beat until well combined.
4. Place 1/4 of the mixture into preheated waffle iron and cook for about 3-4 minutes or until golden brown.
5. Repeat with the remaining mixture.
6. Serve warm.

Nutrition:

- Calories: 158
- Net Carb: 1.4g
- Fat: 14.1g
- Carbohydrates: 2.2g
- Dietary Fiber: 0.8g
- Sugar: 0.5g
- Protein: 4.3g

CREAM CHEESE AND COCONUT OIL CHAFFLES

Servings: 2
Preparation Time: 10 minutes
Cooking Time: 12 minutes

Ingredients:
- 2 ounces cream cheese, softened
- 2 large organic eggs
- 1 tablespoon coconut flour
- 1 tablespoon coconut oil, melted
- ½ teaspoon organic baking powder
- 2-4 drops liquid stevia

Directions:
1. Preheat a mini waffle iron and then grease it.
2. In a bowl, place flour, Erythritol and baking powder and mix well.
3. Add the egg, cream cheese and vanilla extract and beat until well combined.
4. Place 1/4 of the mixture into preheated waffle iron and cook for about 2-3 minutes or until golden brown.
5. Repeat with the remaining mixture.
6. Serve warm.

Nutrition
- Calories: 12 3
- Net Carb: 1.3g
- Fat: 1 lg
- Carbohydrates: 2.1g
- Dietary Fiber: 0.8g
- Sugar: 0.2g
- Protein:4.5g

CREAM LIME PIE CHAFFLE

Serving: 2
Preparation Time: 5 minutes
Cooking Time: 4 minutes

Ingredients:
Chaffle:
- 1 egg
- ¼ cup almond flour
- 2 teaspoons cream cheese, room temperature
- 1 teaspoon Swerve
- ½ teaspoon baking powder
- ½ teaspoon lime extract or 1 teaspoon freshly squeezed lime juice
- ½ teaspoon lime zest
- Pinch of salt

Frosting:
- 4 ounces (113 g) cream cheese, softened
- 4 tablespoons butter
- 2 teaspoons Swerve
- 1 teaspoon lime extract
- ½ teaspoon lime zest

Directions:
1. Preheat the mini waffle maker.
2. Place all the chaffle ingredients in a blender and blend on high until smooth and creamy.
3. With an ice cream scoop and pour in the waffle maker with one full scoop of batter.
4. Cook each chaffle for about 3 to 4 minutes until golden brown.
5. Meanwhile, make the frosting by whisking together all the frosting ingredients in a small bowl until smooth.
6. Let the chaffles cool completely before frosting them.
7. Serve immediately.

Nutrition:
- Calories: 95
- Fat: 5.9g
- Protein: 5.7g

CHEDDAR AND ALMOND FLOUR CHAFFLES

Servings: 2
Preparation time: 10 minutes
Cooking Time: 10 Minutes

Ingredients:
- 1 large organic egg, beaten
- ½ cup Cheddar cheese, shredded
- 2 tablespoons almond flour

Directions:
1. Preheat a mini waffle iron and then grease it.
2. In a bowl, place the egg, Cheddar cheese and almond flour and beat until well combined.
3. Place half of the mixture into preheated waffle iron and cook for about 5 minutes or until golden brown.
4. Repeat with the remaining mixture.
5. Serve warm.

Nutrition:
- Calories: 195
- Net Carb: 1g
- Fat: 15
- Saturated Fat: 7g
- Carbohydrates: 1.8g
- Dietary Fiber: 0.8g
- Sugar: 0.6g
- Protein: 10.2g

CHEDDAR, WHIPPING CREAM AND SUN BUTTER CHAFFILES

Servings: 6
Preparation Time: 0 minutes
Cooking Time: 18 minutes

Ingredients:
- 1/2 cup cheddar cheese, shredded
- 1 organic egg
- 1 organic egg white
- 2 tablespoons heavy whipping cream
- 1 tablespoon sugar-free sun butter
- 2 tablespoons coconut flour
- 3 tablespoons Erythritol
- ¼ teaspoon organic vanilla extract
- 1/8 teaspoon organic baking powder

Directions:
1. Preheat a mini waffle iron and then grease it.
2. In a medium bowl, place all ingredients and with a fork, mix until well combined.
3. Divide the mixture into 6 portions.
4. Place 1 portion of the mixture into pre- heated waffle iron and cook for about 2-3 minutes or until golden brown.
5. Repeat with the remaining mixture.
6. Serve warm.

Nutrition:
- Calories: 95
- Net Carb: 1.4g
- Fat: 7.3g
- Carbohydrates: 2.6g
- Dietary Fiber: 1.2g
- Sugar: 0.4g
- Protein: 5g

CRUNCHY KETO WAFFLES (CHOCOLATE VERSION)

Servings: 2
Preparation time: 15 minutes
Cooking time: 10 minutes

Ingredients:

- 40g low carbohydrate protein powder
- 2 eggs
- 30 g of melted coconut oil
- 50 g pieces of crushed dark chocolate without sugar

Directions:

1. Separate the yolks from the whites and beat the whites with stiff foam.
2. Put the protein powder in a separate bowl, add the melted coconut oil and yolks.
3. Gently add the egg whites, then add the crushed sugar-free chocolate pieces and a pinch of salt.
4. Heat the waffle iron plates and bake the waffles until golden.
5. Adjust the time to achieve a crispy waffle dough.

Nutrition:

- Fat: 30.5 g
- Protein: 27 g
- Net carbohydrates: 9 g
- kcal: 409.5

DELICIOUS RASPBERRIES TACO CHAFFLES

Servings: 1
Cooking Time: 15 minutes

Ingredients:
- 1 egg white
- 1/4 cup jack cheese, shredded
- 1/4 cup cheddar cheese, shredded
- 1 tsp coconut flour
- 1/4 tsp baking powder
- 1/2 tsp stevia

For Topping:
- 4 oz. raspberries
- 2 tbsps. coconut flour
- 2 oz. unsweetened raspberry sauce

Directions:
1. Switch on your round Waffle Maker and grease it with cooking spray once it is hot.
2. Mix together all chaffle Ingredients: in a bowl and combine with a fork.
3. Pour chaffle batter in a preheated maker and close the lid.
4. Roll the taco chaffle around using a kitchen roller, set it aside and allow it to set for a few minutes.
5. Once the taco chaffle is set, remove from the roller.
6. Dip raspberries in sauce and arrange on taco chaffle.
7. Drizzle coconut flour on top.
8. Enjoy raspberries taco chaffle with keto coffee.

Nutrition:
- Protein: 28% 77 kcal
- Fat: 6 187 kcal
- Carbohydrates: 3% 8 kcal.

DOUBLE CHOCOLATE MOZZARELLA AND CREAM CHAFFLES

Servings: 2
Preparation Time: 0 minutes
Cooking Time: 0 minutes

Ingredients:
- 1 organic medium egg
- ½ cup Mozzarella cheese, shredded
- 1 teaspoon double cream
- 2 tablespoons almond flour
- 2 tablespoons cacao powder
- 1 tablespoon 70% dark chocolate chips
- 1 tablespoon granulated Erythritol
- 1 teaspoon organic vanilla extract

Directions:
1. Preheat a mini waffle iron and then grease it.
2. In a bowl, place all ingredients except for chocolate chips and beat until well combined.
3. Gently, fold in the chocolate chips.
4. Place half of the mixture into preheated waffle iron and cook for about 3-4 minutes or until golden brown.
5. Repeat with the remaining mixture.
6. Serve warm.

Nutrition:
- Calories: 174
- Net Carb: 3.2g
- Fat: 13.1g
- Carbohydrates: 6.5g
- Dietary Fiber: 3.3g
- Sugar: 0.7g
- Protein: 6.8g

DOUBLE CHOCO CHAFFLE

Servings: 2
Preparation time: 10 minutes
Cooking Time: 10 Minutes

Ingredients:

- 1 egg
- 2 teaspoons coconut flour
- 2 tablespoons sweetener
- 1 tablespoon cocoa powder
- ¼ teaspoon baking powder
- 1 oz. cream cheese
- ½ teaspoon vanilla
- 1 tablespoon sugar-free chocolate chips

Directions:

1. Put all the ingredients in a large bowl.
2. Mix well.
3. Pour half of the mixture into the waffle maker.
4. Seal the device.
5. Cook for 4 minutes.
6. Uncover and transfer to a plate to cool.
7. Repeat the procedure to make the second chaffle.

Nutrition:

- Calories: 171
- Total Fat: 10.7g
- Saturated Fat: 5.3g
- Cholesterol: 97mg
- Sodium: 106mg
- Potassium: 179mg
- Total Carbohydrate: 3g
- Dietary Fiber: 4.0g
- Protein: 5.8g
- Total Sugars: 0.4g

DOUBLE CHOCOLATE CREAM CHEESE CHAFFLES

Servings: 2
Preparation Time: 10 minutes
Cooking Time: 10 minutes

Ingredients:
- 2 teaspoons coconut flour
- 2 tablespoons Erythritol
- 1 tablespoon cacao powder
- ¼ teaspoon organic baking powder
- 1 organic egg
- 1 ounce cream cheese, softened
- ½ teaspoon organic vanilla extract
- 1 tablespoon 70% dark chocolate chips

Directions:
1. Preheat a mini waffle iron and then grease it.
2. In a bowl, place flour, Erythritol, cacao powder and baking powder and mix well.
3. Add the egg, cream cheese and vanilla extract and beat until well combined.
4. Gently, fold in the chocolate chips.
5. Place half of the mixture into preheated waffle iron and cook for about 5 minutes or until golden brown.
6. Repeat with the remaining mixture.
7. Serve warm.

Nutrition:
- Calories: 151
- Net Carb: 3.1g
- Fat: 11.9g
- Carbohydrates: 5.9g
- Dietary Fiber: 2.8g
- Sugar: 0.3g
- Protein: 5.7g

DOUBLE CHOCOLATE HEAVY CREAM CHAFFLES

Servings: 4
Preparation Time: 10 minutes
Cooking Time: 12 minutes

Ingredients:
- 1 medium organic egg
- 1 tablespoon heavy cream
- 6 tablespoons almond flour
- 2 tablespoons Erythritol
- 1 tablespoon cacao powder
- 2 tablespoons 70% dark chocolate chips
- ¼ teaspoon xanthan gum

Directions:
1. Preheat a mini waffle iron and then grease it.
2. In a bowl, place all ingredients except for chocolate chips and beat until well combined.
3. Gently, fold in the chocolate chips.
4. Place half of the mixture into preheated waffle iron and cook for about 3 minutes or until golden brown.
5. Repeat with the remaining mixture.
6. Serve warm.

Nutrition:
- Calories: 150
- Net Carb: 2.2g
- Fat: 12.4g
- Carbohydrates: 4.9g
- Dietary Fiber: 2.7g
- Sugar: 0.5g
- Protein: 2.7g

EGG-FREE ALMOND FLOUR CHAFFLES

Servings: 2
Preparation time: 10 minutes
Cooking Time: 10 Minutes

Ingredients:

- 2 tablespoons cream cheese, softened
- 1 cup mozzarella cheese, shredded
- 2 tablespoons almond flour 1
- teaspoon organic baking powder

Directions:

1. Preheat a mini waffle iron and then grease it.
2. In a medium bowl, place all ingredients and with a fork, mix until well combined.
3. Place half of the mixture into preheated waffle iron and cook for about 4-5 minutes or until golden brown.
4. Repeat with the remaining mixture.
5. Serve warm.

Nutrition:

- Calories: 77
- Net Carb: 2.4g
- Fat: 9.8g
- Saturated Fat: 4g
- Carbohydrates: 3.2g
- Dietary Fiber: 0.8g
- Sugar: 0.3g
- Protein: 4.8g

Servings: 2
Preparation Time: 10 minutes
Cooking Time: 6 minutes

Ingredients:
1tablespoon ground flaxseed
3 tablespoons water
3 tablespoons almond flour
1tablespoon mayonnaise
1/8 teaspoon organic baking powder

Directions:
1. In a bowl, add flaxseed and water and mix well. Set aside for about 5 minutes.
2. Preheat a mini waffle iron and then grease it.
3. In the bowl of flaxseed mixture, place the remaining ingredients and with a fork, mix until well combined.
4. Place half of the mixture into preheated waffle iron and cook for about 3 minutes or until golden brown.
5. Repeat with the remaining mixture.
6. Serve warm.

Nutrition
- Calories: 115
- Net Carb: 2.7g
- Fat: 9.2g
- Carbohydrates: 4.8g
- Dietary Fiber: 2.1g
- Sugar: 0.9g
- Protein:0.7g

FESTIVE CHAFFLE BREAKFAST CHAFFLE SANDWICH

Servings: 1
Cooking Time:10 Minutes

Ingredients:
- 2 basics cooked chaffles
- Cooking spray
- 2 slices bacon
- 1 egg

Directions:
1. Spray your pan with oil.
2. Place it over medium heat.
3. Cook the bacon until golden and crispy.
4. Put the bacon on top of one chaffle.
5. In the same pan, cook the egg without mixing until the yolk is set.
6. Add the egg on top of the bacon.
7. Top with another chaffle.

Nutrition:
- Calories 5 14
- Total Fat 4 7 g
- Saturated Fat 27 g
- Cholesterol 274 mg
- Sodium 565 mg
- Potassium 106 mg
- Total Carbohydrate 2 g
- Dietary Fiber 1 g
- Protein 21 g
- Total Sugars 1 g

FLUFFY CHOCOLATE CHAFFLES

Serving: 4
Preparation Time: 11 minutes
Cooking Time: 6 minutes

Ingredients:
- 1 large egg
- 1 large egg white
- 2 tablespoons cream cheese
- ½ cup grated Mozzarella cheese
- 2 tablespoons coconut flour
- 2 tablespoons cacao powder
- ½ teaspoon baking powder
- ¼ cup Swerve

Direction
1. Preheat the waffle maker.
2. Place the egg, egg white, cream cheese, and Mozzarella into a blender.
3. Process until smooth. Add the remaining ingredients and process again.
4. Spoon one quarter of the batter into the waffle maker.
5. Cook for 2 to 4 minutes or until golden brown.
6. Transfer the chaffle onto a cooling rack to cool.
7. Repeat with the remaining batter.
8. Serve.

Nutrition:
- Calories: 106
- Fat: 7.1g
- Protein: 7.6g

FLUFFY CHOCOLATE MOUSSE

Servings: 3
Preparation time: 20 minutes
Cooking time: 0 minutes

Ingredients:
- 25 g sugar-free chocolate chips/ dark chocolate
- 240 g cream 36%
- 110 g of cream cheese
- 20 g of powdered erythritol
- 15 g cocoa powder

Directions:
1. In a saucepan, melt the chocolate chips with 60 g of cream over very low heat.
2. In a bowl, beat the cream cheese and erythritol.
3. Then add the melted chocolate chips, cocoa powder and a pinch of salt.
4. Beat until all ingredients combine well.
5. In another bowl, stiffen the remaining 180 g of cream.
6. Serve the chocolate dessert in glasses. Put in layers: chocolate, cream, chocolate, cream.
7. For decoration, the top of the dessert can be sprinkled with chocolate chips or shavings.

Nutrition:
- Fat: 41 g
- Protein: 5.5 g
- Net carbohydrates: 8 g
- kcal: 428

FLUFFY WHITE CHAFFLES

Serving: 4
Preparation Time: 10 minutes
Cooking Time: 7 minutes

Ingredients:
- 1 large egg
- 1 large egg white
- 2 tablespoons cream cheese
- ½ cup grated Mozzarella cheese
- 2 tablespoons coconut flour
- ¼ cup almond flour
- ¼ teaspoon vanilla extract
- ½ teaspoon baking powder
- ¼ cup Swerve

Direction
1. Preheat the waffle maker.
2. Place the egg, egg white, cream cheese, and Mozzarella into a blender.
3. Process until smooth.
4. Add the remaining ingredients and process again.
5. Spoon one quarter of the batter into the waffle maker.
6. Cook for 2 to 4 minutes or until golden brown.
7. Transfer the chaffle into a cooling rack to cool.
8. Repeat with the remaining batter.
9. Serve.

Nutrition:
- Calories: 136
- Fat: 10.0g
- Protein: 8.4g

FRENCH TRADITIONAL CREME BRULEE DESSERT

Servings: 2
Preparation Time: 25 minutes
Cooking Time: 35 minutes

Ingredients:

- 30 g of granular erythritol
- 240 g cream 36%
- 2 egg yolks
- 1 teaspoon of vanilla extract
- pinch of salt

Directions:

1. Set the oven to heat up to 150 ° C.
2. Whip 30 g of erythritol with cream and heat it in a pot over low heat until it dissolves.
3. In a separate container, beat the yolks with the vanilla extract and a pinch of salt until the mass thickens.
4. Pour in the cream slowly and keep stirring.
5. Prepare a casserole dish and two ramekins to put in it. Pour hot water into the bowl until it reaches the middle of the ramekins.
6. Pour the French creme brûlée into the containers and bake for 35 minutes.
7. After removing it, refrigerate it for at least 4 hours.
8. Enjoy the sweet and salty taste!

Nutrition:

- Fat: 49 g
- Protein: 5.75 g
- Net carbohydrates: 4 g
- kcal: 478.5

HEALTHY HOMEMADE MUESLI

Servings: 2
Preparation time: 5 minutes
Cooking time: 5 minutes

Ingredients:
- 1/2 cup of unsweetened coconut flakes
- 60 g of whole or chopped almonds
- 2 tablespoons of chia seeds
- 2 cups of unsweetened almond milk
- 10 drops of liquid stevia - optional

Directions
1. Preheat the oven to 180 degrees and put a baking sheet in it, covered with baking paper with coconut flakes on it.
2. Toast them for five minutes, stirring occasionally to keep them from burning.
3. Combine almonds, chia seeds, roasted coconut flakes and divide into two portions
4. Pour with almond milk.
5. If you want muesli to be sweeter, add a few drops of stevia.
6. Mix and eat for health!

Nutrition:
- Fat: 65% (30 g)
- Protein: 24% (11 g)
- Net carbohydrates: 11% (5 g)
- kcal: 350

HEALTHY LEMON SUGAR-FREE CAKE

Servings: 8
Preparation time: 20 minutes
Cooking time: 45 minutes

Ingredients:
- 1/2 cup of unsalted, melted butter
- 1¾ cup of almond flour
- 1 cup of powder erythritol
- 3 medium lemons
- 3 large eggs

Directions:
1. Mix together the butter, 1 cup of almond flour, 1/4 cup of erythritol and add a pinch of salt.
2. Roll it out evenly and put it into a 20 × 20 cm plate covered with parchment paper.
3. Bake at 175 ° C for 20 minutes.
4. Then let it cool for 10 minutes.
5. In a bowl, mash one of the lemons, then squeeze all 3 lemons, add the eggs, 3/4 cup erythritol, 3/4 cup almond flour and a pinch of salt.
6. Mix the dough filling thoroughly.
7. Pour the filling into the cooled bottom and bake for 25 minutes.
8. Serve the cake decorated with lemon slices and powdered erythritol.
9. Enjoy your meal!

Nutrition:
1. Fat: 75% (26 g)
2. Protein: 17% (8 g)
3. Net carbohydrates: 8% (4 g)
4. kcal:272

HEAVY CREAM CHAFFLES

Servings: 2
Preparation Time: 5 minutes
Cooking Time:4 minutes

Ingredients:
- 1organic egg
- 1tablespoon heavy cream
- 2 tablespoons almond flour
- 1/4 teaspoon organic baking powder
- 1tablespoon Erythritol

Directions:
1. Preheat a mini waffle iron and then grease it.
2. In a medium bowl, place all ingredients and with a fork, mix until well combined.
3. Place half of the mixture into preheated waffle iron and cook for about 3-4 minutes or until golden brown.
4. Repeat with the remaining mixture.
5. Serve warm.

Nutrition:
- Calories: 103
- Net Carb: 1.1 g
- Fat: 8.7g
- Carbohydrates: 1.9g
- Dietary Fiber: 0.8g
- Sugar: 0.4g
- Protein:2.9g

HEAVY CREAM AND PEANUT BUTTER CHAFFLES

Servings: 2
Preparation Time: 5 minutes
Cooking Time: 8 minutes

Ingredients:
- 1 teaspoon coconut flour
- ¼ teaspoon organic baking powder
- 1 organic egg
- 2 tablespoons natural peanut butter
- 1 tablespoon heavy cream
- ½ teaspoon almond extract

Directions:
1. Preheat a mini waffle iron and hen grease it.
2. In a medium bowl, place all ingredients and with a fork, mix until well combined.
3. Place half of the mixture into preheated waffle iron and cook for about 4 minutes or until golden brown.
4. Repeat with the remaining mixture.
5. Serve warm.

Nutrition
- Calories: 166
- Net Carb: 3.2g
- Fat: 13.1g
- Carbohydrates :4.7g
- Dietary Fiber: 1.5g
- Sugar: 1.3g
- Protein: 8.1g

HOMEMADE NUTELLA WITHOUT SUGAR

Servings: 5
Preparation time: 10 minutes
Cooking time: 0 minutes

Ingredients:
- 110 g hazelnuts, preferably roasted
- 30 g cocoa powder
- 15 g of granular erythritol
- 15 g of coconut oil
- 150 g of unsweetened almond milk

Directions:
1. Roast the hazelnuts (if not already baked) on a baking tray in an oven at 180 ° C for about 5 minutes or until lightly golden brown.
2. Add the hazelnuts to a blender and blend until they look like peanut butter.
3. Add cocoa, erythritol, coconut oil and a pinch of salt.
4. Blend again until fully combined.
5. Add the almond milk, mixing between additions.
6. Stop when it reaches a Nutella like consistency.
7. Store in the fridge and enjoy the great taste!

Nutrition:
- Fat: 19 g
- Protein: 5 g
- Net carbohydrates: 5.5g
- kcal: 216

KETO CAKE WITH COCONUT FLAKES

Servings:8
Preparation Time: 10 minutes
Cooking Time:50 minutes

Ingredients:
- 460 g of canned coconut milk
- 30 g of granular erythritol
- 3 eggs
- 30 g of powdered erythritol
- 160 g of coconut flakes

Directions:
1. Pour 230 g coconut milk into a pot and add granulated erythritol, put on medium heat to boil, reduce the heat and stir until the erythritol is dissolved.
2. Cool it down and pour it into the bowl with the egg, powdered erythritol. Blend everything together.
3. Add coconut flakes, the rest of the milk and a little salt.
4. Mix everything well. Put into an oiled dish, put in an oven preheated to 180 °C and bake for 40 minutes, until the coconut keto cake is golden brown.
5. Serve with the shavings sprinkled on.
6. The quick coconut cake is ready.
7. Enjoy your meal!

Nutrition:
- Fat: 27 g
- Protein: 4.9 g
- Net carbohydrates: 3 g
- Kcal: 274

KETO CHEESECAKES WITHOUT CHEESE

Servings: 2
Preparation time: 10 minutes
Cooking time: 30 minutes

Ingredients:
- 170 g of cream cheese
- 5 drops of vanilla extract - optional
- 1 egg
- 10 g of erythritol
- 50 g strawberries, sliced to garnish the cream cheese cheesecake
- 10 g of coconut oil
- 2 g of salt

Directions
1. Blend the cheese with the vanilla extract and a pinch of salt until it is creamy.
2. In a small bowl, beat the egg and slowly
3. Add it to the cheese.
4. Add erythritol, dissolved coconut oil and mix everything together with a mixer.
5. Pour the entire mass into ramekins.
6. Put them in an oven heated to 180°C and leave for 30 minutes if the top will get brown, cover with aluminum foil.
7. The keto cheesecake is the most delicious the next day.
8. Put the sliced strawberries on it and enjoy!

Nutrition:
- Fat: 26 g
- Protein: 8 g
- Net carbohydrates: 5 g
- kcal: 290

KETO CHOCOLATE FUDGE CHAFFLE

Servings: 2
Preparation time: 10 minutes
Cooking Time: 14 Minutes

Ingredients:
- 1 egg, beaten
- ¼ cup finely grated Gruyere cheese
- 2 tbsp unsweetened cocoa powder
- ¼ tsp baking powder
- ¼ tsp vanilla extract
- 2 tbsp erythritol
- 1 tsp almond flour
- 1 tsp heavy whipping cream
- A pinch of salt

Directions:
1. Preheat the waffle iron.
2. Add all the ingredients to a medium bowl and mix well.
3. Open the iron and add half of the mixture.
4. Close and cook until golden brown and crispy, 7 minutes.
5. Remove the chaffle onto a plate and make another with the remaining batter.
6. Cut each chaffle into wedges and serve after.

Nutrition:
- Calories: 173
- Fats: 13.08g
- Carbs: 3.98g
- Net Carbs: 2.28g
- Protein: 12.27g

KETO FUDGY CHOCOLATE CHAFFLES

Serving: 2
Preparation Time: 5 minutes
Cooking Time: 8 minutes

Ingredients:

- 1 egg, beaten
- 2 tablespoons cocoa
- 2 tablespoons shredded Mozzarella cheese
- 2 tablespoons Swerve
- 1 teaspoon heavy whipping cream
- 1 teaspoon coconut flour
- ¼ teaspoon vanilla extract
- ¼ teaspoon baking powder
- Pinch of salt
- Cooking spray

Direction

1. Preheat the waffle maker.
2. Lightly spray it with cooking spray.
3. Mix remaining ingredients then stir to incorporate.
4. Fill in half of the batter into the waffle maker.
5. Close the lid and cook for 4 minutes.
6. Transfer to a plate and repeat with the remaining batter.
7. Serve.

Nutrition:

- Calories: 113
- Fat: 7.3g
- Protein: 7.2g

KETO ICE CREAM: CHOCOLATE MINT ICE CREAM

Servings: 9
Preparation time: 20 minutes
Cooking time: 0 minutes

Ingredients:

- 570 g of unsweetened canned coconut milk
- 2/3 cup of granular erythritol
- 1 medium avocado
- 1/2 teaspoon of mint extract
- 1/2 cup of dark chocolate chips

Preparation:

1. Before starting your recipe, put the drum of the ice cream machine in the freezer and let it sit overnight.
2. In a blender, mix coconut milk, erythritol, avocado, and 1/2 teaspoon of mint extract.
3. Add the chocolate chips.
4. Beat the mixture according to the manufacturer's instructions for the ice cream machine. Put in the freezer overnight.
5. Take it out of the freezer and leave it for 10-15 minutes to gently defrost it and enjoy the ice cream

Tip: Add 1 tablespoon of vodka in step 2 to keep the ice cream soft after freezing.

Nutrition:

- Fat: 78% (18 g)
- Protein: 9% (2 g)
- Net carbohydrates: 13% (3 g)
- kcal: 173

KETO PANCAKES WITH STRAWBERRIES

Servings: 2
Preparation time: 15 minutes
Cooking time: 10 minutes

Ingredients:
- 2 large eggs - separate the yolk from the white
- 2 g baking powder 80 g of crushed strawberries
- 30 g of cream cheese
- 5 drops of vanilla extract optional
- 10 g of coconut oil

Directions:
1. Beat the egg white stiffly with a high-speed electric mixer, at the end add baking powder.
2. Combine the cream cheese, strawberries, yolks so that they have a uniform consistency.
3. Gently mix the strawberry mass with the egg white foam, be careful not to collapse - this is a simple recipe for fluffy pancakes.
4. Pour into a hot, greased pan and fry until the dough is solidified and browned, remembering to turn it over.

Nutrition:
- Fat: 14 g
- Protein: 8 g
- Net carbohydrates: 3 g
- kcal: 170

LEMON POPPY SEED CHAFFLES

Cooking Time: 8 minutes
Serving: 2

Ingredients:
For the chaffles,
- Two tbsp. of almond flour- finely ground
- One tsp. of fresh lemon zest
- One-eighth of tsp. of poppy seeds
- An egg (large-sized)
- A quarter cup of part-skim ricotta cheese
- One tsp. of sugar or any other sweetener you prefer

For the toppings (Optional):
- Fresh berries
- Ricotta cheese

Directions:
1. Take the waffle iron and preheat it.
2. Add ricotta cheese, almond flour, lemon zest, poppy seeds, egg, and sugar in a small bowl.
3. Whisk everything together and let them combine fully.
4. In the preheated waffle iron, drop half a spoon of this mixture.
5. Spread evenly and well.
6. Cook for two to three minutes, or till the smoke starts subsiding
7. Repeat the process with the rest of the batter
8. While serving top with fresh berries and ricotta cheese.
9. Almond flour can be substituted with coconut flour.
10. For two tbsp. of almond flour, two tsps. of coconut flour should be used.
11. After mixing, let the batter sit for ten minutes.
12. This lets the flour absorb the liquid.
13. Refrigerate the chaffles in an airtight container after wrapping them properly.

Nutrition:
- Calories: 231 |
- Carb: 1.56g |
- Protein: 15.2g |

- Fat: 16.7g |
- Fiber: 3g

MACADAMIA NUTS AND PECANS IN CHOCOLATE

Servings: 10
Preparation time: 20 minutes
Cooking time: 0 minutes

Ingredients:
- 1/2 cup of heavy cream
- 50 g of dark chocolate
- 15-20 drops of liquid stevia
- 10 whole pecans
- 20 macadamia nuts

Directions:
1. Heat the fondant cream over low heat (don't let it boil!) And add the finely chopped dark chocolate.
2. Stir until completely dissolved and add some stevia if desired.
3. Arrange 1 pecans and 2 macadamia nuts in 10 small groups on a baking tray lined with parchment paper.
4. Pour or pour about a teaspoon of the chocolate mixture into each nut cluster, covering them completely to keep them all stuck together.
5. Sprinkle each chocolate block with chopped pecans and sea salt, then refrigerate for about 4 hours.

Tip: Bake the nuts for a distinctive flavor!

Nutrition:
- Fat: 79% (9 g)
- Protein: 9% (1 g)
- Net carbohydrates: 11% (1.3 g)
- kcal:100

MAPLE CHAFFLE

Servings: 2
Cooking Time: 15 Minutes

Ingredients:
- 1 egg, lightly beaten
- 2 egg whites
- 1/2 tsp maple extract
- 2 tsp Swerve
- 1/2 tsp baking powder, gluten-free
- 2 tbsp almond milk
- 2 tbsp coconut flour

Directions:
1. Preheat your waffle maker.
2. In a bowl, whip egg whites until stiff peaks form
3. Stir in maple extract, Swerve, baking powder, almond milk, coconut flour, and egg.
4. Spray waffle maker with cooking spray.
5. Pour half batter in the hot waffle maker and cook for 3-minutes or until golden brown.
6. Repeat with the remaining batter.
7. Serve and enjoy.

Nutrition:
- Calories 122
- Fat 6.6 g
- Carbohydrates 9 g
- Sugar 1 g
- Protein 7 g
- Cholesterol 82 mg

MAYONNAISE CHAFFLES

Servings: 2
Preparation Time: 5 minutes
Cooking Time: 10 minutes

Ingredients:
- 1large organic egg, beaten
- 1tablespoon mayonnaise
- 2 tablespoons almond flour
- 1/2 teaspoon organic baking powder
- 1 teaspoon water
- 2-4 drops liquid stevia

Directions:
1. Preheat a mini waffle iron and then grease it.
2. In a medium bowl, place all ingredients and with a fork, mix until well combined.
3. Place half of the mixture into preheated waffle iron and cook for about 4-5 minutes or until golden brown.
4. Repeat with the remaining mixture.
5. Serve warm.

Nutrition
- Calories: 110
- Net Carb: 2.6g
- Carbohydrates: 3.4g
- Dietary
- Fiber: 0.8g
- Sugar: 0.9g
- Protein: 3.2g

MAYONNAISE AND CREAM CHEESE CHAFFLES

Preparation time: 9 minutes
Cooking Time: 20 Minutes
Servings: 2

Ingredients:
- 4 organic eggs large
- 4 tablespoons mayonnaise
- 1 tablespoon almond flour 2
- tablespoons cream cheese, cut into small cubes

Directions:
1. Preheat a waffle iron and then grease it.
2. In a bowl, place the eggs, mayonnaise and almond flour and with a hand mixer, mix until smooth.
3. Place about ¼ of the mixture into preheated waffle iron.
4. Place about ¼ of the cream cheese cubes on top of the mixture evenly and cook for about 5 minutes or until golden brown.
5. Repeat with the remaining mixture and cream cheese cubes.
6. Serve warm.

Nutrition:
- Calories: 190
- Net Carb: 0.6g
- Fat: 17g
- Saturated Fat: 4.2g
- Carbohydrates: 0.8g
- Dietary Fiber: 0.2g
- Sugar: 0.5g
- Protein: 6.7g

MINI BREAKFAST CHAFFLES

Servings:3
Cooking Time: 15 minutes

Ingredients:
- 6 tsp coconut flour
- 1 tsp stevia
- 1/4 tsp baking powder
- 2 eggs
- 3 oz. cream cheese
- 1/2. tsp vanilla extract

For Topping:
- 1 egg
- 6 slice bacon
- 2 oz. Raspberries for Topping
- 2 oz. Blueberries for Topping
- 2 oz. Strawberries for Topping

Directions:
1. Heat up your square waffle maker and grease with cooking spray.
2. Mix together coconut flour, stevia, egg, baking powder, cheese and vanilla in mixing bowl.
3. Pour ½ of Chaffles mixture in a waffle maker.
4. Close the lid and cook the Chaffles for about 3-5 minutes.
5. Meanwhile, fry bacon slices in pan on medium heat for about 2-3 minutes until cooked and transfer them to plate.
6. In the same pan, fry eggs one by one in the leftover grease of bacon.
7. Once Chaffles are cooked, carefully transfer them to plate.
8. Serve with fried eggs and bacon slice and berries on top.
9. Enjoy!

Nutrition:
- Protein: 16% 75 kcal
- Fat: 75% 346 kcal
- Carbohydrates: 9% 41 kcal

MORNING CHAFFLES WITH BERRIES

Servings: 4
Cooking Time: 5 Minutes

Ingredients:
- 1 cup egg whites
- 1 cup cheddar cheese, shredded
- ¼ cup almond flour
- ¼ cup heavy cream

Topping:
- 4 oz. raspberries
- 4 oz. strawberries.
- 1 oz. keto chocolate flakes
- 1 oz. feta cheese.

Directions:
1. Preheat your square waffle maker and grease with cooking spray.
2. Beat egg white in a small bowl with flour.
3. Add shredded cheese to the egg whites and flour mixture and mix well.
4. Add cream and cheese to the egg mixture.
5. Pour Chaffles batter in a waffle maker and close the lid.
6. Cook Chaffles for about 4 minutes until crispy and brown.
7. Carefully remove Chaffles from the maker.
8. Serve with berries, cheese, and chocolate on top.
9. Enjoy!

Nutrition:
- Protein: 28% 68 kcal
- Fat: 67% 163 kcal
- Carbohydrates: 5% 12 kcal

MOZZARELLA AND ALMOND FLOUR CHAFFLES

Servings: 2
Cooking Time: 8 Minutes

Ingredients:
- ½ cup Mozzarella cheese, shredded
- 1 large organic egg
- 2 tablespoons blanched almond flour
- ¼ teaspoon organic baking powder

Directions:
1. Preheat a mini waffle iron and then grease it.
2. In a medium bowl, place all Ingredients: and with a fork, mix until well combined.
3. Place half of the mixture into preheated waffle iron and cook for about 4 minutes or until golden brown.
4. Repeat with the remaining mixture.
5. Serve warm.

Nutrition:
- Calories: 98
- Net Carb: 1.4g
- Fat: 7.1g
- Saturated Fat: 1g
- Carbohydrates: 2.2g
- Dietary Fiber: 0.8g
- Sugar: 0.2g Protein: 7g

MOZZARELLA AND BUTTER CHAFFLES

Servings: 2
Preparation Time: 10 minutes
Cooking Time: 8 minutes

Ingredients:
- 1large organic egg, beaten
- ¾ cup Mozzarella cheese, shredded
- ½ tablespoon unsalted butter, melted
- 2 tablespoons blanched almond flour
- 2 tablespoons Erythritol
- ½ teaspoon ground cinnamon
- ½ teaspoon Psyllium husk powder
- ¼ teaspoon organic baking powder
- ½ teaspoon organic vanilla extract

Directions:
1. Preheat a waffle iron and then grease it.
2. In a medium bowl, place all ingredients and with a fork, mix until well combined.
3. Place half of the mixture into preheated waffle iron and cook for about 3-5 minutes or until golden brown.
4. Repeat with the remaining mixture.
5. Serve warm.

Nutrition
- Calories: 140
- Net Carb: 1.9g
- Fat: 10.6g
- Carbohydrates: 3g
- Dietary Fiber: 1.1g
- Sugar: 0.3g
- Protein: 7.8g

MOZZARELLA AND CREAM CHEESE CHAFFLES

Servings: 2
Preparation Time: 10 minutes
Cooking Time: 8 minutes

Ingredients:
- 1 organic egg, beaten
- 1 tablespoon cream cheese, softened
- ½ cup Mozzarella cheese
- 1tablespoon Erythritol
- ¼ teaspoon organic vanilla extract
- ¼ teaspoon organic almond extract

Directions:
1. Preheat a waffle iron and then grease it.
2. In a medium bowl, place all ingredients and with a fork, mix until well combined.
3. Place half of the mixture into preheated waffle iron and cook for about 3-4 minutes or until golden brown.
4. Repeat with the remaining mixture.
5. Serve warm.

Nutrition
- Calories: 124
- Net Carb: 6.6g
- Fat: 10.2g
- Carbohydrates: 1g
- Dietary Sugar: 0.5g
- Protein: 9.4g

MOZZARELLA PEANUT BUTTER CHAFLLES

Servings: 2
Preparation Time: 5 minutes
Cooking Time: 8 minutes

Ingredients:
- 1 organic egg, beaten
- ½ cup Mozzarella cheese, shredded
- 3 tablespoons granulated Erythritol
- 2 tablespoons peanut butter

Directions:
1. Preheat a mini waffle iron and then grease it.
2. In a medium bowl, place all ingredients and with a fork, mix until well combined.
3. Place half of the mixture into preheated waffle iron and cook for about 4 minutes or until golden brown.
4. Repeat with the remaining mixture.
5. Serve warm.

Nutrition
- Calories: 145
- Net Carb: 2.6g
- Fat: 11 g
- Carbohydrates: 3.6g
- Dietary Fiber: 1g
- Sugar: 1.7g
- Protein: 8.8g

MOZZARELLA AND YOGURT CHAFFLES

Servings: 2
Preparation Time: 10 minutes
Cooking Time: 8 minutes

Ingredients:
- ½ cup Mozzarella cheese, shredded finely
- 1 tablespoon plain Greek yogurt
- 1 organic egg
- 2 tablespoons ground almonds
- ½ teaspoon psyllium husk
- ¼ teaspoon organic baking powder
- 2-3 drops liquid stevia

Directions:
1. Preheat a mini waffle iron and then grease it.
2. In a medium bowl, place all ingredients and with a fork, mix until well combined.
3. Place half of the mixture into preheated waffle iron and cook for about 3-4 minutes or until golden brown.
4. Repeat with the remaining mixture.
5. Serve warm.

Nutrition
- Calories: 93
- Net Carb: 1.7g F
- at: 6.7g
- Carbohydrates: 2.8g
- Dietary Fiber: 1.1g
- Sugar: 0.8g
- Protein: 6.3g

MOZZARELLA AND XANTHAN GUM CHAFFLES

Servings: 2
Preparation Time: 5 minutes
Cooking Time: 8 minutes

Ingredients:
- ¼ cup blanched almond flour
- 2 tablespoons powdered Erythritol
- Pinch of xanthan gum
- ½ cup Mozzarella cheese, shredded
- 1 large organic egg

Directions:
1. Preheat a waffle iron and then grease it.
2. In a medium bowl, place all ingredients and with a fork, mix until well combined.
3. Place half of the mixture into preheated waffle iron and cook for about 3-4 minutes or until golden brown.
4. Repeat with the remaining mixture.
5. Serve warm.

Nutrition
- Calories: 146
- Net Carb: 1.4g
- Fat: 11.2g
- Carbohydrates: 2.9g
- Dietary Fiber: 1.5g
- Sugar: 0.7g
- Protein: 5.2g

NUTTY BANANA CHAFFLES

Serving: 2
Preparation Time: 5 minutes
Cooking Time: 8 minutes

Ingredients:
- 1 egg
- ½ cup Mozzarella cheese
- 1 tablespoon cream cheese, softened
- 1 tablespoon Swerve, plus more for serving
- ¼ teaspoon sugar-free banana extract
- ¼ teaspoon vanilla extract
- Chopped pecans, for serving

Directions:
1. Preheat the mini waffle maker.
2. Whip the egg in a small bowl.
3. Stir in remaining ingredients and stir until well incorporated.
4. Pour half the batter into the waffle maker and cook for a minimum of 4 minutes until golden brown.
5. Transfer to a plate and repeat with the remaining batter.
6. Serve topped with the Swerve and pecans.

Nutrition
- Calories: 116
- Fat: 7.9g
- Protein: 8.9g

PEANUT BUTTER CHAFFLE

Preparation Time: 5 minutes
Cooking Time: 8 minutes
Serving: 2

Ingredients:
- 1 egg, beaten
- ½ cup shredded Mozzarella cheese
- 3 tablespoons Swerve
- 2 tablespoons peanut butter

Direction
1. Preheat the waffle maker.
2. Incorporate all the ingredients then stir until well incorporated.
3. Fill in half of the batter into the waffle maker and cook for 4 minutes.
4. Transfer to a plate to cool.
5. The chaffle will be a little flimsy when you remove it, but it will stiffen up as it cools.
6. Repeat with the remaining batter.
7. Serve warm.

Nutritions Value
- Calories: 213
- Fat: 16.3g
- Protein: 13g

PEANUT BUTTER AND JELLY CHAFFLES

Servings: 1
Preparation Time: 5 minutes
Cooking Time: 15 minutes

Ingredients:
- 1 egg
- 2 slices cheese, thinly sliced
- 1 tsp natural peanut butter
- 1 tsp sugar-free raspberry
- Cooking spray

Directions:
1. Crack and whisk the egg in a small bowl or a measuring cup.
2. Lightly grease the waffle maker with Cooking spray.
3. Preheat the waffle maker.
4. Once it is heated up, place a slice of cheese on the waffle maker and wait for it to melt.
5. Once melted, pour the egg mixture onto the melted cheese.
6. Once the egg starts cooking, carefully place another slice of cheese on the waffle maker.
7. Close the lid. Cook for 3-4 minutes.
8. Take out the Chaffles and place on a plate.
9. Top the Chaffles with whipped cream.
10. Drizzle some natural peanut butter and raspberry on top.

Nutrition:

- Calories: 337
- Cal Total Fat: 27 g
- Saturated Fat: 0 g
- Cholesterol: 0 mg
- Sodium: 0 mg
- Total Carbs: 3 g
- Fiber: 0 g
- Sugar: 0 g
- Protein: 21 g

PROTEIN CREAM CHEESE CHAFFLES

Servings: 6
Preparation Time: 10 minutes
Cooking Time: 30 minutes

Ingredients:
- 1 organic egg
- 1 tablespoon Erythritol
- 1 teaspoon ground cinnamon
- ¼ cup cream cheese, softened
- 2 tablespoons almond flour
- 1 tablespoon unsweetened protein powder
- ½ teaspoon organic baking powder
- ½ teaspoon organic vanilla extract

Directions:
1. Preheat a mini waffle iron and then grease it.
2. In a bowl, add egg, Erythritol and cinnamon and with a hand mixer, mix until fluffy.
3. Add the remaining ingredients and mix until well combined.
4. Divide the mixture into 6portions.
5. Add 1portion into preheated waffle iron and cook for about 3-5 minutes or until golden brown.
6. Repeat with the remaining mixture.
7. Serve warm.

Nutrition
- Calories: 62
- Net Carb:0.8g
- Fat: 5.4g
- Carbohydrates: 1.3g
- Dietary Fiber:0.5g
- Sugar: 0.2g
- Protein: 2.6g

PROTEIN MOZZARELLA CHAFFLES

Servings:4
Preparation Time: 10 minutes
Cooking Time: 20 minutes

Ingredients:
- ½ scoop unsweetened protein powder
- 2 large organic eggs
- ½ cup Mozzarella cheese, shredded
- 1 tablespoon Erythritol
- ¼ teaspoon organic vanilla extract

Directions:
1. Preheat a mini waffle iron and then grease it.
2. In a medium bowl, place all ingredients and with a fork, mix until well combined.
3. Place ¼ of the mixture into preheated waffle iron and cook for about 4-5 minutes or until golden brown.
4. Repeat with the remaining mixture.
5. Serve warm.

Nutrition
- Calories: 61
- Net Carb:0.4g
- Fat: 3.3g
- Carbohydrates: 0.4g
- Sugar: 0.2g
- Protein: 7.3g

PROTEIN MOZZARELLA AND CREAM CHEESE CHAFFLES

Servings: 3
Preparation Time: 10 minutes
Cooking Time: 15 minutes

Ingredients:
- 1 ounce cream cheese, softened
- ½ cup Mozzarella cheese, shredded
- 2 tablespoons unflavored whey protein isolate
- 2 tablespoons powdered Erythritol
- ½ teaspoon organic baking powder
- 1 organic egg
- ½ teaspoon organic vanilla extract

Directions:
1. Preheat a mini waffle iron and then grease it.
2. In a microwave-safe bowl, add cream cheese and Mozzarella cheese and microwave for about 1-1 ½ minutes or until the cheeses are melted, stirring after every 30 seconds.
3. Remove from the
4. Add the whey protein, Erythritol and baking powder and with your hands, knead until well combined.
5. Add the egg and vanilla extract and beat until smooth.
6. Add 1/3 of the mixture into preheated waffle iron and cook for about 3-5 minutes or until golden brown.
7. Repeat with the remaining mixture.
8. Serve warm.

Nutrition
- Calories: 142
- Net Carb: 6.6g
- Fat: 10.1g
- Carbohydrates: 1.5g

PUDDING WITH PEANUT BUTTER AND COCOA BEANS

Servings: 2
Preparation time: 5 minutes
Cooking time: 12 hours

Ingredients:

- 300 g of unsweetened almond milk
- 30 g of chia seeds
- 50 g of peanut (or almond) butter
- 5 drops of liquid stevia (optional)
- 20 g cocoa beans

Preparation:

1. In the evening, combine almond milk, chia seeds, peanut butter and liquid stevia in a large bowl.
2. Mix everything until you get the right consistency (the peanut butter must blend well with the rest of the ingredients, so you can mix it in a blender).
3. Transfer the mixture to the dish where you will serve it and cover it with cling film.
4. Set aside in the refrigerator overnight.
5. In the morning, sprinkle the top of the dish with cocoa beans.
6. Enjoy your meal!

Nutrition:

- Fat: 34 g
- Protein: 14.5 g
- Net carbohydrates: 2.3 g
- kcal: 410

PUMPKIN-CINNAMON CHURRO STICKS

Preparation time: 10 minutes
Cooking Time: 14 Minutes
Servings: 2

Ingredients:
- 3 tbsp coconut flour
- ¼ cup pumpkin puree
- 1 egg, beaten
- ½ cup finely grated mozzarella cheese
- 2 tbsp sugar-free maple syrup + more for serving
- 1 tsp baking powder
- 1 tsp vanilla extract
- ½ tsp pumpkin spice seasoning
- 1/8 tsp salt
- 1 tbsp cinnamon powder

Directions:
1. Preheat the waffle iron.
2. Mix all the ingredients in a medium bowl until well combined.
3. Open the iron and add half of the mixture.
4. Close and cook until golden brown and crispy, 7 minutes.
5. Remove the Chaffle onto a plate and make 1 more with the remaining batter.
6. Cut each Chaffle into sticks, drizzle the top with more maple syrup and serve after.

Nutrition:
- Calories: 219
- Fats: 9.72g
- Carbs: 8.g
- Net Carbs: 4.34g
- Protein: 25.27g

PUMPKIN AND PECAN CHAFFLE

Preparation time: 10 minutes
Cooking Time: 10 Minutes
Servings: 2

Ingredients:

- 1 egg, beaten
- ½ cup mozzarella cheese, grated
- ½ teaspoon pumpkin spice
- 1 tablespoon pureed pumpkin
- 2 tablespoons almond flour
- 1 teaspoon sweetener
- 2 tablespoons pecans, chopped

Directions:

1. Turn on the waffle maker.
2. Beat the egg in a bowl.
3. Stir in the rest of the ingredients.
4. Pour half of the mixture into the device.
5. Seal the lid. Cook for 5 minutes.
6. Remove the Chaffle carefully.
7. Repeat the steps to make the second Chaffle.

Nutrition:

- Calories 210
- Total Fat 17 g
- Saturated Fat 10g
- Cholesterol 110 mg
- Sodium 250 mg
- Potassium 570 mg
- Total Carbohydrate 4.6 g
- Dietary Fiber 1.7 g
- Protein 11 g
- Total Sugars 2 g 15.

RASPBERRY CHAFFLES

Servings: 2
Prep Time: 5 minutes
Cook Time: 6 minutes

Ingredients
- 4 Tbsp almond flour
- 4 large eggs
- 2 ⅓ cup shredded mozzarella cheese
- 1 tsp vanilla extract
- 1 Tbsp erythritol sweetener
- 1½ tsp baking powder
- ½ cup raspberries

Directions
1. Turn on waffle maker to heat and oil it with cooking spray.
2. Mix almond flour, sweetener, and baking powder in a bowl.
3. Add cheese, eggs, and vanilla extract, and mix until well-combined.
4. Add 1 portion of batter to waffle maker and spread it evenly.
5. Close and cook for 3-4 minutes, or until golden.
6. Repeat until remaining batter is used.
7. Serve with raspberries.

Nutritional Value (per serving):
- Calories: 303
- Fat: 11 g
- Carbohydrate: 5g
- Protein: 22g

RASPBERRY PORRIDGE ON VEGETABLE MILK

Servings: 2
Preparation time: 5 minutes
Cooking time: 8 minutes

Ingredients:
- 400 g of unsweetened coconut milk
- 20 g coconut shavings
- 20 g of ground linseed
- 60 g of raspberries
- 100 g of water
- optional: 6 drops of liquid stevia

Directions
1. Heat the coconut milk with water in a small saucepan.
2. When the milk begins to evaporate, add ground flaxseed and coconut shavings to it.
3. Mix all ingredients thoroughly.
4. Add the raspberries and cook until thickened.
5. Raspberries should tint the porridge a beautiful pink color.
6. You can optionally blend the entire porridge. If you like sweet porridge, add stevia to it and it's ready!

Nutrition:
- Fat: 49 g
- Protein: 6 g
- Net carbohydrates: 9 g
- kcal: 504

RASPBERRY KETO SHORTBREAD COOKIES

Servings:8
Preparation Time: 15 minutes
Cooking Time: 15 minutes

Ingredients:
- 120 g of cream cheese
- 1 egg
- 40 g of erythritol powder
- 115 g of almond flour

Directions:
1. Start making the keto cookie dough by mixing half the cream cheese with 30 g of erythritol, egg, almond flour and a pinch of salt.
2. In the second bowl, prepare the biscuit filling by mixing the remaining cheese and 10 g of erythritol.
3. In another bowl, blend raspberries with a tablespoon of erythritol.
4. On a baking tray lined with baking paper, form small cookies, on top of them put the mass from the other bowl, and on top of the blended raspberries.
5. Bake for 15 minutes in an oven preheated to 175 ° C. Once cooled down, eat some delicious keto cookies.
6. Enjoy your meal!

Nutrition:
- Fat: 78% (30 g)
- Protein: 9% (3.5 g)
- Net carbohydrates: 13% (5 g)
- kcal: 300

RED VELVET CREAM CHAFFLES

Servings: 2
Preparation Time: 10 minutes
Cooking Time: 8 minutes

Ingredients:
- 2 tablespoons cacao powder
- 2 tablespoons Erythritol
- 1 organic egg, beaten
- 2 drops super red food coloring
- ¼ teaspoon organic baking powder
- 1 tablespoon heavy whipping cream

Directions:
1. Preheat a mini waffle iron and then grease it.
2. In a medium bowl, add all ingredients and with a fork, mix until well combined.
3. Place half of the mixture into preheated waffle iron and cook for about 4 minutes.
4. Repeat with the remaining mixture.
5. Serve warm.

Nutrition:
- Calories: 70
- Net Carb: 1.7g
- Fat: 6g
- Carbohydrates: 3.2g
- Dietary Fiber: 1.5g
- Sugar: 0.2g
- Protein: 3.9g 69)

RED VELVET CREAM CHEESE CHAFFLES

Servings: 4
Preparation Time: 10 minutes
Cooking Time: 10 minutes

Ingredients:
- 2 organic eggs
- 2 ounces cream cheese, softened
- 2 tablespoons unsweetened almond milk
- ¼ cup coconut flour
- 1½ tablespoons Erythritol
- 1 teaspoon organic baking powder
- ½ teaspoon cacao powder
- 2-3 drops red food coloring

Directions:
1. Preheat a mini waffle iron and then grease it.
2. In a medium bowl, add all ingredients and with a fork, mix until well combined.
3. Place ¼ of the mixture into preheated waffle iron and cook for about 3-5 minutes.
4. Repeat with the remaining mixture.
5. Serve warm.

Nutritional Information
- Calories: 114
- Net Carb: 3.2g
- Fat: 4.3g
- Carbohydrates: 6.3g
- Dietary Fiber: 3.1g
- Sugar: 0.2g
- Protein: 4.9g

SLIMMING COCKTAIL WITH COCONUT MILK AND MACADAMIA NUTS

Servings: 1
Preparation time: 5 minutes
Cooking time: 0 minutes

Ingredients:
- 2 cups of unsweetened coconut milk
- 30 g of macadamia nuts
- 1/4 cup unsweetened coconut flakes
- 1/2 teaspoon of ground cinnamon
- 10 drops of liquid stevia

Directions:
1. Put all ingredients in a blender and blend until creamy.
2. Sweeten with stevia to taste. If you don't like its taste, you can replace it with erythritol.
3. Serve cold.

Nutrition:
- Fat: 84% (38 g)
- Protein: 7% (3 g)
- Net carbohydrates: 9% (4 g)
- kcal: 390

STRAWBERRY SHORTCAKE CHAFFLE BOWLS

Preparation time: 15 minutes
Cooking Time: 28 Minutes
Servings: 2

Ingredients:
- 1 egg, beaten
- ½ cup finely grated mozzarella cheese
- 1 tbsp almond flour
- ¼ tsp baking powder
- 2 drops cake batter extract
- 1 cup cream cheese, softened
- 1 cup fresh strawberries, sliced
- 1 tbsp sugar-free maple syrup

Directions:
1. Preheat a waffle bowl maker and grease lightly with cooking spray.
2. Meanwhile, in a medium bowl, whisk all the ingredients except the cream cheese and strawberries.
3. Open the iron, pour in half of the mixture, cover, and cook until crispy, 6 to 7 minutes.
4. Remove the chaffle bowl onto a plate and set aside.
5. Make a second chaffle bowl with the remaining batter.
6. To serve, divide the cream cheese into the chaffle bowls and top with the strawberries.
7. Drizzle the filling with the maple syrup.
8. Serve.

Nutrition:
- Calories 235
- Fats 20.62g
- Carbs 5.9g
- Net Carbs 5g
- Protein 7.51g 13.

SWISS CHEESE AND YOGURT CHAFFLES

Servings: 2
Preparation Time: 10 minutes
Cooking Time: 10 minutes

Ingredients:
- 1 large organic egg
- 1 tablespoon full-fat Greek yogurt
- 1 tablespoon almond flour
- 1/8 teaspoon organic baking powder
- 2-4 drops liquid stevia
- ¼ cup Swiss cheese, shredded

Directions:
1. Preheat a waffle iron and then grease it.
2. In a bowl, add eggs, yogurt, flour, baking powder and stevia and beat until well combined.
3. Place ¼ of cheese into preheated waffle iron and top with half of egg mixture.
4. Sprinkle with ¼ of cheese.
5. Repeat with the remaining cheese and egg mixture.
6. Serve warm.

Nutrition
- Calories: 115
- Net Carb: 1.8g
- Fat: 8.2g
- Carbohydrates: 2.2g
- Dietary Fiber: 0.4g
- Sugar: 1g
- Protein: 7.2g

SWEET POTATO CRANBERRY CHAFFLES

Servings: 5
Cooking Time: 25 minutes

Ingredients:
For the chaffles,
- One and a half cup of sweet potato puree
- Two tbsp. of shredded mozzarella
- Two tbsp. of brown sugar
- An egg (slightly beaten)
- One-eighth tsp. of ground cloves
- One-fourth tsp. of ground nutmeg
- One tsp. of ground cinnamon
- One and a half cups of all-purpose flour
- One and a half tbsp. of baking powder
- A quarter tsp. of ground ginger
- One-eight tsp. of salt

For the syrup:
- Half a cup of cranberry sauce
- A cup of maple syrup
- Half a tsp. of ground cinnamon

Directions:
1. Start with preheating the waffle iron.
2. Stick to the instruction manual from the manufacturer for this process.
3. In a bowl, add sweet potato puree, egg, and shredded mozzarella.
4. Stir and mix together.
5. In another large bowl, add baking powder, brown sugar, one tsp. of cinnamon, flour, ginger, cloves, nutmeg powder, and salt.
6. Whisk everything together.
7. Now mix the contents of both bowls.
8. Combine the batter together by stirring.
9. Now, in the waffle iron, drop the batter with a ladle.
10. The chaffles should completely turn crisp and golden.
11. Cook for three minutes to get this result.
12. In a saucepan, mix maple syrup, half a tsp. of cinnamon, and cranberry sauce, and heat in medium flame.

13. Stir the content occasionally.
14. They should be well heated and combined thoroughly.
15. This can take around five to ten minutes.
16. Take off the cooked chaffles and transfer them to a plate.
17. Pour the syrup on the chaffles.
18. Use aluminum foil for cooking the chaffles evenly, and for keeping it moist.
19. It can also help in making the cleaning process easy.

Nutrition:
- Calories: 517
- Carbs: 108.2g
- Protein: 7.9g
- Fat: 7g
- Fiber: 3g

VANILLA CREAM CHEESE CHAFFLES

Servings: 2
Preparation Time: 10 minutes
Cooking Time: 8 minutes

Ingredients:
- 2 teaspoons coconut flour
- 3 teaspoons Erythritol
- 1/4 teaspoon organic baking powder
- 1 organic egg
- 1ounce cream cheese, softened
- 112 teaspoon organic vanilla extract

Directions:
1. Preheat a mini waffle iron and then grease it.
2. In a bowl place flour, Erythritol and baking powder and mix well.
3. Add the egg, cream cheese and vanilla extract and beat until well combined.
4. Place half of the mixture into preheated waffle iron and cook for about 3-4 minutes or until golden brown.
5. Repeat with the remaining mixture.
6. Serve warm.

Nutrition:
- Calories:95
- Net Carb: 1.6g
- Fat: 7.4g
- Carbohydrates: 2.6g
- Dietary Fiber: 1g
- Sugar: 0.3g
- Protein:4.2g

VANILLA HEAVY CREAM CHAFLLES

Servings: 2
Preparation Time: 5 minutes
Cooking Time: 6 minutes

Ingredients:
- 6 tablespoons almond flour
- 1/4 teaspoon xanthan gum
- 2 tablespoons Erythritol
- 1medium organic egg
- 1tablespoon heavy cream
- 1teaspoon organic vanilla essence

Directions:
1. Preheat a mini waffle iron and then grease it.
2. In a medium bowl, place all ingredients and with a fork, mix until well combined.
3. Place half of the mixture into preheated waffle iron and cook far about 2-3 minutes or until golden brown.
4. Repeat with the remaining mixture.
5. Serve warm.

Nutrition:
- Calories: 200
- Net Carb: 2.1g
- Fat: 16.2g
- Carbohydrates: 4.8g
- Dietary Fiber: 2.7g
- Sugar: 1.2g
- Protein:2.9g

VANILLA MOZZARELLA CHAFFLES

Servings: 2
Preparation Time: 10 minutes
Cooking Time: 12 Minutes

Ingredients:

- 1 organic egg, beaten
- 1 teaspoon organic vanilla extract
- 1 tablespoon almond flour
- 1 teaspoon organic baking powder
- Pinch of ground cinnamon
- 1 cup Mozzarella cheese, shredded

Directions:

1. Preheat a mini waffle iron and then grease it.
2. In a bowl, place the egg and vanilla extract and beat until well combined.
3. Add the flour, baking powder and cinnamon and mix well.
4. Add the Mozzarella cheese and stir to combine.
5. In a small bowl, place the egg and Mozzarella cheese and stir to combine.
6. Place half of the mixture into preheated waffle iron and cook for about 5-minutes or until golden brown.
7. Repeat with the remaining mixture.
8. Serve warm.

Nutrition:

- Calories: 103
- Net Carb: 2.4g
- Fat: 6.6g
- Saturated Fat: 2.3g
- Carbohydrates: 2
- Dietary Fiber: 0.5g
- Sugar: 0.6g
- Protein: 6.8g

NOTES

....

....

....

....

....

....

....

....

....

....

....

....

....

....

....

....

....

....

....

....

....

....

CPSIA information can be obtained
at www.ICGtesting.com
Printed in the USA
BVHW012112260321
603406BV00016B/129